ESSENTIAL LAW AND E... IN NURSING

T0092744

This thoroughly updated third edition lays a solid foundation for understanding the intersection of law, ethics and the rights of the patient in the context of everyday nursing and health care practice.

Outlining the key legal and ethical principles relevant to nurses, *Essential Law and Ethics In Nursing: Patients, Rights and Decision-Making*, previously entitled *Patients' Rights: Law and Ethics for Nurses,* uses an easy-to-read style that conveys key principles in an accessible way. It:

- provides a clear understanding not only of basic legal provisions in health care but also of wider issues relating to human rights;
- covers topics such as ethical decision-making, the regulation of nursing, confidentiality, laws concerning human rights, safe practice, vulnerable people, elder abuse and employment regulations; and
- includes thinking points, case studies and relevant case law to help link theory with practice.

This is essential reading for nurses and an important reference for midwives and allied health professionals.

Paul Buka, MSc (Leic.), PGCE, LL.B (Hons) (Law), FETC (City and Guilds, 7307), HNC (Public Admin law), RN, RNT, ENB 998, ENB 923, MIHM, FHEA, Member of the Institute of Medical Ethics, is lecturer in Adult Nursing at the University of Essex, UK, specialising in healthcare law and ethics. Previously senior lecturer and Programme Lead (Overseas Nursing Programme) at the University of West London, UK. Paul undertook his nurse training in Fife, Scotland, specialising in Trauma and Orthopaedics, with clinical experience in Care of older people, Acute Medicine, Trauma and Orthopaedics and Mental Health. As a ward manager, Paul developed a keen interest in legal studies. He read law at Higher National Certificate, degree and postgraduate levels. He was keen to share with others his specialist interest (in Healthcare Law and Ethics, human rights of vulnerable people) through writing for publication, given the limited texts, on the market at the time which were suitable for students. He started teaching law in Further Education at ILEX Diploma level and subsequently Healthcare Law and Ethics in Higher Education from undergraduate to post-registration/graduate levels. He also gained experience in teaching other aspects of nurse education. Paul has authored and co-authored previous publications in this area.

ESSENTIAL LAW AND ETHICS IN NURSING

Patients, Rights and Decision-Making

Third Edition

Paul Buka

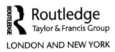

Routledge
Taylor & Francis Group

LONDON AND NEW YORK

Third edition published 2020
by Routledge
2 Park Square, Milton Park, Abingdon, Oxon, OX14 4RN

and by Routledge
52 Vanderbilt Avenue, New York, NY 10017

Routledge is an imprint of the Taylor & Francis Group, an informa business

© 2020 Paul Buka

The right of Paul Buka to be identified as author of this work has been asserted by him in accordance with sections 77 and 78 of the Copyright, Designs and Patents Act 1988.

All rights reserved. No part of this book may be reprinted or reproduced or utilised in any form or by any electronic, mechanical, or other means, now known or hereafter invented, including photocopying and recording, or in any information storage or retrieval system, without permission in writing from the publishers.

Trademark notice: Product or corporate names may be trademarks or registered trademarks, and are used only for identification and explanation without intent to infringe.

First edition published by Hodder Arnold 2008
Second published by Routledge 2014

British Library Cataloguing-in-Publication Data
A catalogue record for this book is available from the British Library

Library of Congress Cataloging-in-Publication Data
Names: Buka, Paul, author.
Title: Essential law and ethics in nursing: patients, rights and decision-making / Paul Buka.
Description: Third edition. | Abingdon, Oxon; New York, NY: Routledge, 2020. | Includes bibliographical references and index. |
Summary: "This thoroughly updated third edition lays a solid foundation for understanding the intersection of law, ethics and the rights of the patient, in the context of everyday nursing and health care practice"—Provided by publisher.
Identifiers: LCCN 2020011545 (print) | LCCN 2020011546 (ebook) | ISBN 9780367262440 (hardback) | ISBN 9780367262457 (paperback) | ISBN 9780429292187 (ebook)
Subjects: LCSH: Nursing—Law and legislation—Great Britain. | Nursing ethics—Great Britain. | Patients—Legal status, laws, etc.—Great Britain.
Classification: LCC KD2968.N8 .B85 2020 (print) | LCC KD2968.N8 (ebook) | DDC 344.4104/14—dc23
LC record available at https://lccn.loc.gov/2020011545
LC ebook record available at https://lccn.loc.gov/2020011546

ISBN: 978-0-367-26244-0 (hbk)
ISBN: 978-0-367-26245-7 (pbk)
ISBN: 978-0-429-29218-7 (ebk)

Typeset in Times New Roman
by codeMantra

To Carol, my wife, my family; Alannah and Sandy (Mummy and Daddy), George; Joshua and Hana, our delightful grandchildren and my extended family. Thank you for putting up with me and for all your support in the development of this project.

Contents

Boxes

Foreword

It is a great honour to have been invited to write the foreword for the third edition of the book titled *Essential Law and Ethics In Nursing: Patients, Rights and Decision-Making*.

Every single nurse needs to ensure that their practice is safe, accountable and based on the most up-to-date evidence. This entails having a sound grasp of the ethical theories, principles and frameworks used within our legislative and professional frameworks. These are necessary to protect and uphold our human rights as citizens and professionals, safeguarding us from unnecessary harm or violation of our rights and dignity. Possessing this legal and ethical knowledge is imperative because we are living and working in a world that is exceptionally busy, fast-moving and evolving almost daily.

Globalization, commercialization and consumerism are affecting every sphere of health care, and nursing is not immune or impervious to these challenges and forces. The net effect is that each of us as members of the public and potential users of health care has high expectations with regard to the quality and outcome of our encounters with healthcare providers and professionals.

Needless to say, the delivery of health care is complex and multifaceted, and it is delivered within a range of settings, such as home, hospital and urban and rural environments. Nursing as a profession is integral and fundamental to the provision of compassionate, person-centred health care. At the heart of all nursing is ensuring we support the essential, holistic needs of our patients (physical, psychological, social, spiritual), who come from diverse cultures and ethnic backgrounds. Each person possesses their own unique worldview, which will undoubtedly have been nurtured through beliefs, values, attitudes and practices, some of which may have been passed down across many generations or acquired through distinct and sometimes difficult life experiences or situations.

When I reflect upon the nurse of today, they are very different from the nurse of yesterday; the landscape of nursing and our societies have changed significantly. There is greater emphasis placed on interdisciplinary and partnership working. Some of the skills, tasks and duties once performed by doctors have been devolved and undertaken by nurses in a variety of clinical settings. While this role explanation is welcome it does pose a greater risk to the nurse because of the potential for a blurring of boundaries. This means that the nurse needs to be more informed, ensuring that they practise within acceptable protocols and frameworks: for example, a nurse prescriber adhering to the correct formulary.

Similarly, when one reflects upon the patient of today, their needs have become far more complex and acute, requiring intense support and interventions. For example, babies who are born prematurely have an increased chance of survival, and their lives are sustained and preserved through new technologies. Meanwhile life expectancy has increased significantly for many of us, necessitating nurses caring for and supporting many 'extreme' older people with advanced frailty, multiple co-morbidities and complex needs. Nurses are confronted with far more complex ethical challenges and decisions around life and death, placing greater emphasis on the need to have sound knowledge to ensure that they always act in the best interest of their patients while not compromising their own ethical values and position.

Furthermore, nursing education in many countries is now provided within Higher Education Institutions, reinforcing the fact that a greater emphasis is placed on knowledge, skills and attitudes in order to practice competently and safely. There is greater awareness of the need for inclusion and equality in order to prevent any form of discrimination or abuse.

Interestingly, while the roles and responsibilities of nursing have changed the essentials of nursing have remained constant: for example, ensuring that everyone is treated with dignity and respect across the lifespan continuum. Contemporary nursing and health care have certainly evolved, and the public's expectations of what is acceptable has heightened. This may be in part due to greater and rapid access to information through the internet and social media. The outcome is that members of the public are far more informed today about their own human and legal rights and are very proactive in ensuring that these are met and upheld. Rightly so! We all want the best and highest standards of care for ourselves and family members.

Therefore, I wholeheartedly endorse and recommend this updated third edition, which considers new case law and legal frameworks. The text provides a valuable and accessible introduction into some of the key, often-complex aspects of legal and ethical issues. This has been achieved successfully through a combination of reflection and interactive exercises. The use of scenarios and cases helps to illustrate different case law, raising awareness of key ethical and legal principles for nurses supporting their learning. The outcome is a very useful text that will enable the nurse of today and tomorrow to practice safely and crucially in accordance with the standards and Codes of Professional Regulatory bodies. The text gives the reader a step-by-step navigation through the changing landscape of legal, ethical issues while informing them about the human and legal rights of their patients and the professional obligations that this involves.

Professor Wilfred McSherry
Professor in Nursing
Department of Nursing
School of Health and Social Care
Staffordshire University
University Hospitals of North Midlands NHS Trust
Part time Professor VID University College, Norway

Preface

Service users of today should be able to feel empowered and informed about their care. This third edition will also focus on informing the nurse as a healthcare provider on rights in a caring context. Service users and lay carers may also find it useful.

With improved technology and quality of healthcare provision, more people are living. The European Convention on Human Rights Act 1950 was enacted (in the United Kingdom) by passing the Human Rights Act 1998. This clearly defined human rights within a patient-centred relationship. Nurses are also becoming more autonomous and accountable. Expectations of safe provision of health care are inevitable, with increased complaints and litigation. Nurses owe service users, a duty of care in ethics and law, and should recognize this, safeguarding those who are at risk. Aspects of current policy are engaged, and ethical principles are the basis for professional conduct as they are linked to every patient's fundamental rights; the law should take precedence.

This book does not purport to have all the answers. This should be the domain of a standard comprehensive legal textbook. Rather, it aims to provide an introduction and application of a bioethical and legal framework within which care should be delivered. It could be argued that ethics informs the law and regulates the conduct of citizens and healthcare professionals. Key aspects of the law herein are based on United Kingdom law, though they are applicable to comparable systems. The author recognizes that, wherever possible, every effort will be made to highlight key distinctions between English and Scots law, with occasionally limited application to Northern Ireland. Due to the nature and size of this book, a comprehensive and detailed analysis would not be practical.

In healthcare provision, 'formal' codes of professional conduct have been drawn based on law and bioethics. Gone are the days when the nurse would hope to evade prosecution or litigation based on paternalism or the grounds that they were following 'the doctor's orders'. With an advanced scope of practice comes a higher level of accountability. It is hoped that by challenging nurses to raise awareness of the legal and ethical implications of their decisions and actions, the quality of care they provide can be improved. Knowledge and application of legal and ethical principles is necessary for understanding and defining patients' rights putting them at the centre of clinical decision-making.

Acknowledgements

I am grateful to Grace McInnes, senior publishing editor, Joanna Koster, senior publisher, for the first edition and to Evie Lonsdale, publishing assistant, all at Taylor and Francis; for their guidance and support and, to Jeanine Furino, Project manager and the production team at Codemantra, without whom this project would not have been possible. Many thanks to Professor Wilfred McSherry for kindly providing a foreword for this edition.

To Jim Sumpter and Ed Holt, both lecturers at the University of Essex (UoE); Cheyne Truman, a final-year BSc Adult Nursing student at UoE; Laura Carlin, staff nurse at the Royal Victoria Hospital, Dundee, Scotland; and last, but not least, Rob Clark, nurse practitioner in rheumatology at Kings College University Hospital, London, and a post-registration student at UoE – thank you all very much for your patience and for the painstaking chapter reviews while trying to make sense of drafts. All your suggestions were constructive and invaluable. This is much appreciated.

Not forgetting all my wonderful colleagues in the team for the School of Health and Social Care (University of Essex), who I have not named, for the kindness and valued support you showed during a traumatic and personally difficult time for me in the past few months. I am especially indebted to the adult nursing team, the mental health nursing team and the administrative staff at the Southend Campus.

Finally, a big thank you to all the students I am privileged to have worked with over the years; for all the informal feedback on previous publications. I do not forget the most important people, those we cared for, who were service users. As healthcare professionals, we are honoured to have been privy to their individual patient journeys.

Introducing ethics in health care

Chapter outline

Introduction and overview

The aim of this chapter is to introduce the key concepts of ethics while applying them to health care. Ethical principles emerged from a variety of systems of moral principles which influenced thinking and decision-making for moral philosophers or ethicists. These principles may apply to a range of aspects or situations in people's lives, from the beginning of life to the end. Ethics or moral philosophy attempts to define norms of how people should live while providing a forum on what these standards should be. There are many variations of ethics theories, and they serve as guiding principles in a variety of settings and help decision-makers in distinguishing right from wrong. The question remains how to determine the most appropriate interventions for supporting decision-making in a given healthcare setting. There are many theories which attempt to provide some answers. Due to the nature and complexity of treatment decisions, application of ethical principles presents a challenge when competing interests may emerge, and tensions of human conflict may be exposed. Ethics may lend a hand in providing some answers. Ethical values may be at variance with other principles such as those based on law, for example, in the interpretation of statutes as informed by case law. In the provision of care, the service-user should be at the centre of decision-making (NHS Constitution, 2015). Within the wider society, applied ethical standards may regulate the conduct of groups of non-healthcare professionals such as architects, lawyers, tradesmen and other professionals. Nurses and midwives also fall into this category via the Nursing and Midwifery Council (NMC). Ethics is concerned with decisions affecting individuals and how the impact of family, friends and society. Ethics is often described as a branch of philosophy: namely 'moral philosophy'. The discipline has evolved from a variety of sources with factors in any given society and includes the following moral choices on:

- how to live a good life
- our rights and responsibilities
- the language of right and wrong
- moral decisions – what is good and bad?

(http://www.bbc.co.uk/ethics/introduction/intro_1.shtml)

The word 'ethics' ('εθιks) originates from the Greek 'ethos'. The branch of moral philosophy, ethics or sometimes loosely termed 'morals', may develop from societal norms of human conduct, which have shaped specific standards of conduct to which various professions of various disciplines subscribe. The Greek philosophers who were credited with developing moral philosophy were Socrates (c. 470–399 BCE), Plato (429?–347 BCE) and Aristotle (384–322 BC).

Stoicism

The 'Stoics' followed a prominent school founded by Zeno of Citium in Cyprus (344–262 BCE) and were responsible for the revival of Plato and Aristotle's 'Virtue Ethics'.

They built philosophy of life based on positive aspects and maximizing positive emotions based on practical ways to help improve a person's strength of character. They also focussed on a person's morals, character or the individual's integrity. Some examples are very broad, and they include honesty, courage, fairness and compassion. Could this be part of a person's individual integrity or 'conscience', both of which can be described as innate or rather as acquired later in life as the individual chooses to act in the way they do? The Stoics also identified *wisdom, justice, fortitude* and *temperance* as the 'four cardinal virtues'; these are found within Plato's *Republic*.

Moral philosophy or ethics classification may also be sub-divided into four approaches or sub- topics:

- Meta-ethics aims to understand the nature of ethical evaluations, the origin of ethical principles and the meanings of terms used but is value-free.
- Descriptive ethics involves, for example, determining what proportion of the population or a certain group considers that something is right or wrong.
- Normative ethics, sometimes referred to as moral theory, focusses on how moral values are determined, what makes things right or wrong and what should be done.
- Applied ethics examines controversial issues (such as euthanasia, abortion and capital punishment) and applies ethical theories to real-life situations. Applied ethical issues are those which are clearly moral issues and for which there are significant groups of people who are either for or against.

(https://www.alzheimer-europe.org/Ethics/Definitions-and-approaches/
What-is-meant-by-the-term-ethics)

The discipline of applied ethics is relevant to healthcare practice when it comes to clinical decision-making.

Key ethical theories

The issue is, whether a claim that those universal ethical principles with common ground for morals which are acceptable to the majority of a given society can be justifiable. What should happen when a conflict of morals arises, and whose morality is it, anyway? Norms vary, from society to society, groups to groups or between individuals. Ethics usually revolves around distinguishing good from bad or right from wrong. Ethical dilemmas may arise in health care, and ethical principles may be invoked in support of viewpoints during decision-making, thus resolving disputes. The relation to the law will be demonstrated. It is possible that in one society it may be difficult to guarantee individual rights to choose where treatment decisions arise. Where decision-making involves several stakeholders, it may be difficult to have a consensus on a given ethical theory as morals or by norms for distinguishing right from wrong. It could be argued that ethical norms are relative to nations or individuals, depending on the society in which they have been brought up. It may be possible to hold that individuals born and bred within the same family, who are brought up within the same environment and under the same conditions, such as circle of friends, religion, schooling and neighbourhood, may later in life hold divergent ethical values. There are exceptions to the rule of morals when 'unethical' conduct may be acceptable in some sub-cultures such as those found in criminal fraternities. Hence the question remains whether there can ever be a consensus of universally accepted norms of ethics. Alongside other branches of philosophy, ethics or moral philosophy has evolved over centuries. Many ethical theories have both similarities and divergent ideas on the interpretation of what is ethical, that is, distinguishing right from wrong.

Although ethics can be described as a system of moral principles or rules, it is not quite an accurate reflection of ethics as there are different approaches to defining ethics. There are, however, some core ethical principles which are universally accepted. The development of ethical values may be linked to religion, culture and customs, while others have developed international treaties. There is no simplistic answer as to what is or is not acceptable, and this goes beyond responses to the dilemma between good and bad. The two main categories of ethical theories are consequentialism and non-consequentialism.

Virtue ethics

Greek moral philosophers are credited with originating ethical theories. The 'triumvirate' of moral philosophy in ancient Greece society was Socrates (470/469–399 BC), Plato (428–347 BC) and Aristotle (384–322 BC), who were largely accredited with developing moral philosophy or ethics as a discipline.

Socrates (470/469–399 BC) was hailed as not only the father of democracy but also the founder of virtue ethics which was followed by the Stoics. This was based on his questioning method. Virtue ethics was based on character traits or moral character rather than ethical duties, responsibility including the most basic of ethics, beneficence, non-maleficence and autonomy. Bioethical ethics developed from these principles (below).

Consequentialism

Consequentialism is concerned with outcomes or results of any action as a justification such as the greatest good for the greatest number. Teleology, which is a branch of consequentialism, may judge actions to be 'right 'or 'wrong' based on their consequences.

Another branch of consequentialism is utilitarianism, which judges the morality of actions based on their utility or usefulness. The more prominent proponents of utilitarianism were Jeremy Bentham (1748–1832) and John Stuart Mill (1806–73). They broadly agreed that actions are morally right when they produce the most good (greatest happiness) for the majority of people (for the greatest number).

They were hedonistic in their approach, though against an egocentric (individual-focussed approach. This is maximization of benefits of a majoritarian theory which may have a problem in justifying overriding the rights of minorities, for example in respect of older people with multiple conditions, or whether seeking treatment for a small number of people with rare conditions. Consider whether the outcome or greater good be the deciding factor in allocation of resources. This could also mean excluding life-changing treatment for a small number of people who require substantial amounts of resources. The so-called Postcode Lottery has also been linked to consequentialism and unequal distribution of resources.

There are two branches: act utilitarianism and rule utilitarianism.

a. *Act utilitarianism* – An act is considered right if it results in a positive and good outcome. Alternative for the greatest number.
b. *Rule utilitarianism* – An act is right if and only if it is determined by a rule which belongs to a set of rules; these would lead to a greater good for society, the best possible option.

Both branches of utilitarianism judge the ethics of rightfulness of an act based on its consequences for the greatest number. The limitation of utilitarianism is that one cannot necessarily predict the outcome or consequences of any action; hence, the anticipated consequence may be wrong and therefore not a valid basis for decision-making. Such a reason-based approach to determine decision-making could not be justified.

Non-consequentialism (the main branch is deontology)

There were several ethicists who followed this school of thought, though it had many versions. The most famous branch is deontology, introduced by Immanuel Kant (1724–1804), one of the philosophers who developed the 'categorical imperative', which was based on an internal sense of 'duty' requiring an individual to act. The actor must 'obey', and this is based on reason. One example is that it would be wrong to tell a lie for saving a friend from a murderer. Individuals have a duty to do the right thing (such as tell the truth) regardless of consequences. The difficulty with this theory is that the sense of 'duty' may be relative to individuals and subjective, without fully explaining where the sense of duty comes from. The premise of the argument for an innate sense of duty is weak. Again, one fundamental problem with both these moral schools of thought is that their basis for the justification of their decision-making appears to be flawed.

The emergence of a bioethical theory

Patients are likely to be vulnerable due to illness. The human interaction presents the challenge of a relationship between the patient and a clinician, which is based on trust, a fiduciary relationship. There is an imbalance. Ethical issues may arise as this caring relationship is unequal and based on trust which may be exploited. The medical model empowered doctors and nurses while potentially compromising patients' human rights by making decisions about their treatment. Bioethics emerged in due course as applied ethics associated with medicine was adopted by allied healthcare professions. Ethical principles were integrated into their own codes of conduct and professional ethics. At times when treatment decisions are made, a dilemma or conflict of interest related to morality or different options may arise in decision-making. In ethical decision-making, there may be room for deliberation and compromise (Beauchamp and Childress, 2013).

A patient-centred care focus, NHS Constitution (2015), should be based on ethical values. This means that healthcare models are expected to plan and deliver care, with values such as principlism (the four principles) including patient autonomy. This becomes even more significant because patients are now more empowered and informed about their human rights.

Early medicine was guided by the development of the Hippocratic Oath, though taking this is no longer a requirement for medical practitioners. The ethical perspective is clear towards the end of the oath.

The Hippocratic Oath, (Ορκος)
... So long as I maintain this Oath faithfully and without corruption, may it be granted to me to partake of life fully and the practice of my art, gaining the respect of all men for all time. However, should I transgress this Oath and violate it, may the opposite be my fate.

(Translated by Michael North, National Library of Medicine, 2002)

The Oath of Hippocrates (400 BC) is probably the most famous code of ethics, in ancient medicine. Since the emergence of medicine as a discipline, bioethical principles developed alongside moral philosophy with universal variations. These have common values for many professional medical or healthcare cultures. These were subsequently adopted by professional codes of conduct for medical professions in different countries, over time. With regard to the question 'Who does bioethics (sometimes called biomedical ethics) apply to?' this suggests that it is not only doctors but all allied healthcare professionals, including nurses. Such professionals are expected to be guided by bioethics which are integrated into their professional codes which regulate professional conduct. Professional bodies are bound by their own professional codes of conduct, and these have been drawn up, incorporating the key ethical principles.

Ancient history has shown that medical ethics was developed from or alongside classical ethical theories, from the early days of medicine as a profession. It is clearly the case that as far back as the '3rd Dynasty' in Egypt practising surgery for eyes and teeth considered the relevance of applied ethics. A surgeon looking after a patient was required to treat but recognize the limitations of their knowledge and skills, and what was ethical conduct.

A. "Until he recovers."
B. "Until the period of his injury passes by."
C. "Until thou knowest that he has reached decisive point."

(Third Dynasty [Egypt, 2700 BCE])

A thousand years later came the emergence of Hammurabi's Managed Health Care – circa 1700 BC – which offered some guidance on remuneration for doctors or surgeons. This would not carry the same weight as modern-day damages in a clinical negligence claim against a healthcare professional.

§218 If a physician operate on a man for a severe wound with a bronze lancet and cause the man's death, or open an abscess in the eye of a man with a bronze lancet and destroy the man's eye, they shall cut off his fingers.

§219–220 If a physician operate on the slave of a freeman for a severe wound with a bronze lancet and cause his death, he shall restore a slave of equal value. If he open an abscess in his eye with a bronze lancet, and destroy his eye, he shall pay silver to the extent of one-half his price (average prices for male slaves ranged from 16–30 shekels).

(https://www.managedcaremag.com/archives/1997/5/
hammurabis-managed-health-care-circa-1700-bc)

The Physician's Oath emerged after the Second World War, and international medical codes have adopted most of the ethical values for the healthcare professional.

At the time of being admitted as a member of the medical profession:

- I solemnly pledge myself to consecrate my life to the service of humanity;
- I will give to my teachers the respect and gratitude which is their due;
- I will practice my profession with conscience and dignity; the health of my patient will be my first consideration;
- I will maintain by all the means in my power, the honor and the noble traditions of the medical profession; my colleagues will be my brothers;
- I will not permit considerations of religion, nationality, race, party politics or social standing to intervene between my duty and my patient;
- I will maintain the utmost respect for human life from the time of conception, even under threat, I will not use my medical knowledge contrary to the laws of humanity;
- I make these promises solemnly, freely and upon my honor.

(Declaration of Geneva, 1948)

How healthcare professionals should follow ethical rules should not be determined by 'a gut feeling'; rather they should follow bioethical principles. It is difficult to justify following one's conscience alone as healthcare professionals are bound by their individual professional codes of conduct. Bioethical principles serve as a framework for how we care for patients and in decision-making; *prima facie* (on the face of it), they should be followed by the healthcare professionals until or unless they conflict with other rules, such as their professional codes or relevant legal policy frameworks. In reaching clinical decisions, there can be conflicts between law and ethics; this will be explored below.

Gillon (1994) was one of the pioneers in adapting and applying ethics to health care. This arose in the form of bioethical principles in the United Kingdom. This focussed on Principlism (the four principles), which included beneficence, non-maleficence, autonomy and justice. In implementing treatment decisions, healthcare professionals may look to a framework and should be informed by their professional codes of conduct for guidance based on 'a framework of moral norms'. Principlism is one such framework which is commonly applied in medicine. These principles are closely related to the Seedhouse Grid, Freegard (2007), and this puts ethics at the centre of decision-making in complex situations.

> The term "Principlism" designates an approach to biomedical ethics that uses a framework of ethical principles that are both basic and global in application. Principlist theory concentrates on the philosophical and practical roles that these principles should play in bioethics
>
> (Beauchamp and Rauprich, 2015)

Bioethical principles come in four main principles, with professional codes of conduct adopting the key elements of ethics from which Principlism developed. Bioethical principles apply to all medical and allied health professionals who care for people in the healthcare environment. Regulatory bodies have adopted Principlism (Beauchamp and Childress, 2013) and are recognized as pioneers in the United States.

Beneficence – the first of these principles encompasses the importance of promoting a positive approach to actively doing good for advocating and promoting a service user's welfare. The aim of treatment interventions should be the promotion of human rights and/or maximizing the patient's welfare for those affected by their scope of practice. This is relevant for the person. In research involving clinical trials, the welfare of the participants must be paramount. There is a sense of a moral duty to act in this regard.

Non-maleficence – this may be described as the other side of the coin, like the Hippocratic Oath, the 'do no harm' principle. It is often the case that, in respect of specific clinical interventions, including personal care, recipients of the service are more likely to remember the negative aspects than the positive aspects which they received. The emphasis of the principle applies to the concept of avoiding harm, not inflicting it on a patient, when you deliver care. In Tort Law, this is the basis of duty of care, and negligence is a result of omission rather than commission. One example is omission through neglect. This includes risk assessments and risk management while minimizing harm, Buka (2015). Care delivery should consider the negative aspects including negligence through omission or neglect.

Autonomy – this is an ethical principle which recognizes the right of a person with mental capacity or competency to make an informed choice. This means that for valid consent an important element is competency or capacity to make informed decisions. Capacity or competence can be determined by assessment, which is linked to the five key principles of the Mental Capacity Act 2005. This right to freedom is guaranteed under the Human Rights Act 1998. The relevant aspect is:

> Article 8 – Right to respect for private and family life, which safeguards an individuals' right to make an informed choice? Autonomy gives the patient, the rights to accept or refuse treatment except as provided for by the law. Exceptions are under the Mental Health Act 1983, Public law in control of epidemiology or in emergencies. A person may also be deprived of their liberties under article 5 of the European Convention on Human Rights 1950. The nurse must facilitate the decision-making process for a patient who has capacity. Where a person lacks capacity, stakeholders must act in the patient's best interests. This principle also

applies in emergency cases. The person's right to choose is not absolute. This may be limited where the rights of others may be encroached or where there are safety issues, a patient who lacks mental capacity may have their rights legally infringed by deprivation of their liberty in the interest of safety, Article 5, Human Rights 1998.

Justice or fairness – this applies the principle of fair distribution of scarce resources. In addition, it applies to fairness and non-discriminatory treatment of individual or group rights. This is now linked to the Article 14 of the Human Rights Act 1998 as well as the Equality Act 2010. This principle may cause some difficulty if this is seen to promote equal treatment for all. In fact, it is not possible to treat everyone the same. The aim should be to treat everyone according to their needs, which are diverse. The teleological theories attempt to address the need for fair distribution of resources. It is difficult to justify an action by the result or maximization of the greatest number of people.

Development of professional regulation (NMC) and ethics

The link between ethics and professional regulation will be explored. Following the medical model, paternalism had been justified as the norm, though this was not nec- essarily justifiable. This meant that a patient had no autonomy and they trusted the doctor to make treatment decisions which were in their best interest (Beauchamp and Childress, 2013). Healthcare professionals including nurses and midwives were not val- ued and considered to be 'handmaids' of the doctor. This perception started to change through empowerment of nurses during the Crimean War (1853–56) by pioneers such as Florence Nightingale (1820–1910) and Mary Seacole (1805–81). Both women helped to change the perception of a subservient nursing profession, with a focus on ethical values based on virtue ethics, non-maleficence and compassion. 'It may seem a strange principle to enunciate as the very first requirement in a hospital that it should do the sick no harm', said Florence Nightingale (1863).

Today's nurses are more autonomous. With autonomy comes accountability; hence the need for the development of nursing ethics. There is more focus on the character or conduct of nurses as professionals: how does nurses' conduct outside the workplace affect their professional status?

Box 1.1 Thinking point

J., a deputy ward manager, suspects that G., her ward manager, may be misusing al- cohol. This seems to happen following each payday and is also evident from her poor timekeeping and more frequent lateness for work. Occasionally J has smelt of alcohol in the morning. She has been noticed leaving work early. Other staff have not noticed any problems. There has so far been no evidence of a direct impact on patient care. G. explains to J. in confidence that she has been facing personal issues and stress as her partner is having an affair, and the relationship is in tatters.

What action should J. take?

History shows that nursing and midwifery took some time to establish a regulatory body independent of the medical profession which followed ethical values and a professional code developing what has come to be known as nursing ethics. Globally, the nursing profession for itself an International Council for Nurses first adopted the Code of Ethics for Nurses in 1953. This was revised in 2012. This a federation of 120 nursing professional associations such as the Royal College of Nursing (UK). It also aimed to provide some guidance for nurses in daily management of evidence-based practice and consideration of ethical dilemmas.

- PREAMBLE Nurses have four fundamental responsibilities: to promote health, to prevent illness, to restore health and to alleviate suffering. The need for nursing is universal. Inherent in nursing is a respect for human rights, including cultural rights, the right to life and choice, to dignity and to be treated with respect.
- Nursing care is respectful of and unrestricted by considerations of age, colour, creed, culture, disability or illness, gender, sexual orientation, nationality, politics, race or social status.

(https://www.icn.ch/)

The purpose of establishing a professional regulatory body was safeguarding and protecting the public. Until 1979 the General Nursing Council was the regulatory body for nursing and midwifery. The Briggs Report on Nursing 1972 had recommended changes for the nurse training to improve accountability. This would also mean the establishment of one statutory body with responsibility for regulating education and training of nurses and midwives. The United Kingdom Central Council for Nursing (UKCC) was formed in 1983, bonding the regulation in Scotland, Northern Ireland and Wales. This has since been named as the Nursing and Midwifery Council 2002.

1. The Nursing and Midwifery Council (NMC) is the regulatory body for nursing midwifery and health visiting. Established by Parliament, and with a UK-wide remit, the Council's primary purpose is to protect the public. It achieves this through maintaining a register of nurses, midwives and health visitors, through setting and monitoring standards of education, practice and conduct, and through handling complaints about misconduct and unfitness to practise of those on the register.
2. The NMC was established under the Nursing and Midwifery Order 2001 and opened for business on 1 April 2002. The first Council is a transitional one and, as such, has been wholly appointed by the government

(https://publications.parliament.uk/pa/ld200304/ldselect/ldconst/68/68we53.
htmernment)

It is one matter for professional codes of conduct to adopt ethical values and quite another for them to implement and protect the public (the 6 Cs NHS, 2012). This is a challenge which regulatory bodies have faced as demonstrated by the Morecambe Bay Investigation Report which found that

3. ... a combination of poor clinical skills and knowledge, lack of engagement, lack of ownership of problems, and failure to escalate concerns amongst maternity staff led to problems not being evident at Trust level. Governance systems

were not sensitive enough to identify this problem in the absence of other indicators of poor outcome prior to 2008.

and

4. Had the clinical problems been escalated effectively to more senior level prior to 2008, it is possible that effective corrective action could have been taken before the dysfunctional nature of the unit that we have described elsewhere became embedded and more widespread.

(Report of the Morecambe Bay Investigation, 2015)

The NMC Code (2018) incorporates the bioethical principles.

Ethical dilemmas and framework for decision-making

In reaching treatment decisions, it is vital that they are justified and patient-centred in approach (NHS Constitution, 2015). It is never straightforward to make decisions for people with multiple and complex needs When working within a team of healthcare MDT of professionals, there may be a divergence of opinions on treatment options. Differences of views on benefit to be derived for the patient, vis-à-vis stakeholders, such as healthcare staff and family members, may also arise. This is also possible when a person lacks capacity. Divergencies may also arise due to religious, cultural or social background. When some issues arise, ethics is not always able to provide an answer, only some guidance.

Bioethical principles have a place in decision-making in that they point decision-makers in the right direction, but they do not necessarily provide an automatic solution.

Box 1.2 Thinking point

Mr Y. is an 89-year-old retired army colonel who had been self-caring with minimum assistance until his admission from residential care to A&E one winter morning. He has been diagnosed with exacerbation of COPD and pneumonia. He has also a known diagnosis of early signs of dementia, and he has been treated for mild depression following the death of his wife one year ago. Mr Y. is mentally alert. The hospital is under pressure for beds due to winter pressure. The on-call consultant physician is overheard talking to the registrar saying, 'the old fogey is finished with no chance of recovery. We should not waste resources as we need the beds for younger patients'. He recommends IV antibiotics for 24 hours, then discharging him back to the residential care home for palliative care, regardless of his condition. There was nothing more they could do as the hospital has a bed crisis. The son and daughter, and the patient had not been involved in decision-making. They are upset when they overhear the plan as this is also within their father's earshot. They are adamant that he should be admitted and monitored in hospital as he did well with a similar bout of infection the previous winter. They contact the CQC to complain about what they see as insensitive, ageist and discriminatory treatment of older people in an acute hospital.

1   What are the ethical issues arising here?
2   What course of action would you recommend?

NICE guidelines recommend that healthcare professionals work with patients in decision-making. An ethical approach should consider the following principles apply assuming the patient has mental capacity.

Application of the Seedhouse grid aims to improve a multi-disciplinary and partnership (with patient) approach as well as the opportunity for reflecting on the choices before them. The patient and healthcare staff can consider the options and related information. This should enable the patient to make an informed choice. This also allows healthcare professionals to apply ethical bioethical principles as well as a duty of candour and openness. The process should focus on patient-centred decision-making (NHS Constitution, 2015), summarizing the following key points:

- The patient is informed of all treatment options, explaining the benefits as well as the risks of the treatment.
- The patient is made aware of any realistic choices available to them, and given time to fully explore and weigh these and make a choice without influence or pressure from the healthcare professional or their family.
- A decision is reached working in partnership with a health and social care professional.

The partnership with the patient may be a difficult one considering the need for a fair distribution of limited resources, especially with a winter bed crisis. This often means striking a balance between the patient's needs and other competing factors, putting them at the centre of decision-making.

> The Ethical Grid is a tool, and nothing more than that .... The Grid can enhance deliberation- it can throw light into unseen corners and can suggest new avenues of thought – but it is not a substitute for personal judgement.
>
> (Seedhouse, 1998, p. 209)

The nurse must also respect a patient's (who has mental capacity) decision even if this appears to be an irrational or 'unwise' or 'foolish' decision. Where the patient lacks capacity decisions must be made in the patient's best interests. The bioethical principles (Principlism) underpin the professional codes of conduct including the NMC Code (2018):

Seedhouse criticized Principlism and put forward his own alternative grid building in additional safeguards for the patient in decision-making. Like the NHS Constitution (2015) the focus should be on patient-centred care (Seedhouse, 2009). In bioethics, Principlism or the Four Principles is nevertheless still widely applied in healthcare provision.

Ethics and research

Social science and medical research ethics developed alongside bioethics. In the advancement of medicine, there was a need for research to benefit patients rather than dubious, pointless and unethical experimental research. The establishment of research ethics committees means that any research including human subject is subject to approval. There is otherwise a danger that human rights could be abused by exposing human subjects to extreme or dangerous conditions and substances, all in the name of research. During the two World Wars, it emerged that vulnerable people were being abused and tortured. The abuse got out of control and participants died as a result of injuries related to Nazi Human Experimentation, in the name of experimental research. The so-called 'experiments' centred on three topics: survival of military personnel, testing of drugs and treatments, and the advancement of Nazi racial and ideological goals (Holocaust Encyclopaedia, 2019). One disturbing aspect aimed at cleansing the population of Germany. The choice of victims was discriminatory, mainly on grounds of ethnicity, targeting an estimated population of 6 million Jews as well as others. These included Protestants; Catholics; Poles; Russians; Roma Gypsies; and people with physical disabilities, learning needs and mental health illness, and discriminated on the grounds of sexual orientation (Berenbaum, 2006).

The Nuremberg Code (1947) was formulated in response to the need to reinforce ethics in experimental research, identifying the need for justice for victims of the atrocities perpetrated by the Nazis. Consent should be at the heart of research in order to safeguard participants, though there are exceptions.

> The duty and responsibility for ascertaining the quality of the consent rests upon each individual who initiates, directs or engages in the experiment. It is a personal duty and responsibility which may not be delegated to another with impunity.
>
> (Nuremberg Code, 1949)

The Nuremberg Doctors' Trials lasted for 140 days and ended with the prosecution of 23 German doctors who had taken part in the so-called Nazi 'research' programme. Between September 1939 and April 1945, they had conducted experiments on people regarded to have an unworthy life. These experiments could result in euthanasia. According to the indictments, experiments included the following:

- High-Altitude Experiments
- Freezing Experiments
- Malaria Experiments
- Lost (Mustard) Gas Experiments
- Sulfanilamide Experiments
- Bone, Muscle, and Nerve Regeneration and Bone Transplantation Experiments
- Sea-Water Experiments
- Epidemic Jaundice Experiments
- Sterilization Experiments
- Spotted Fever (Fleckfieber) Experiments
- Experiments with Poison
- Incendiary Bomb Experiments

(https://www.famous-trials.com/nuremberg/1903-doctortrial)

The Nuremberg Trials (1903) indicted perpetrators under international law auspices and found a verdict of 'guilty' for 16 of the doctors, of whom 7 were sentenced to death. The Nuremberg Code (1947) was followed by the Declaration of Helsinki (1964). This was adopted by the World Medical Assembly (revised in 1975). More recently, the

Economic and Social Research Council (ESRC) (2006) was developed to safeguard participants; it was updated again in 2012. The elements of consent should include:

- Competence of participants
- Adequate information
- Consent is given voluntarily

(Florence Nightingale, 1863)

The Universal Declaration of Human Rights 1945 was an international treaty in response to the Second World War abuses of human rights. This was founded on moral philosophy. The Belmont Report (1979) was influential in re-enforcing the need for ethical considerations, including the three principles, respect for persons, beneficence and justice. This was designed to maximize the safety of human participants as well as to avoid harm. Other ethical principles which may define research ethics include respect for privacy, anonymity and confidentiality with respect to any information which the researcher acquires during the research process. The issues of information and data protection will be addressed in Chapter 4.

Conclusion

Gone are the days of paternalism and domineering of passive patients by paternalistic doctors. Ethical theories developed a range of principles which continue to define standards and offer alternative courses of action in every walk of life. Rather than providing answers to every question ethics can be useful as a guiding tool for working through dilemmas and providing options. The development of moral philosophy or ethics goes back to the beginnings of Western civilization and philosophy. This was evolved from local customs, cultures and religions in instilling values which regulate human conduct, by trying to show the way people should conduct themselves in respect of interactions with other human beings. Today, there may be tensions between ethics and the legal framework. The impact of ethics on health care should not be underestimated, and the application of ethics to healthcare has had a huge impact. The development of bioethics has affected the way in which nurses and healthcare professionals care for patients and how patients also perceive their rights. Bioethics aims to define and improve the relationship between patients, healthcare staff and other carers.

References

Alzheimer – Europe., Personhood, Available online at: https://www.alzheimer-europe.org/ Ethics/Definitions-and-approaches/What-is-meant-by-the-term-ethics (accessed on 19th July 2019).

Alzheimer's Society, Ethics Definitions and Approaches. Available online at: https://www. alzheimer-europe.org/Ethics/Definitions-and-approaches/What-is-meant-by-the-term-ethics (accessed on 20th June 2019).

BBC, Ethics: a general introduction. Available online at: http://www.bbc.co.uk/ethics/introduction/ intro_1.shtml (accessed on 20th July 2019).

Beauchamp TL and Childress JF. *Principles of biomedical ethics*, 7th ed. Oxford and New York: Oxford University Press, 2013.

Beauchamp TL and Rauprich O. *Principlism, encyclopaedia of global bioethics*, doi:10.1007/978-3-319-05544-2_348-1, 2015.

Berenbaum M. *The world must know: The history of the Holocaust as told in the United States Holocaust Memorial, Liverpool Museum*, revised ed. Baltimore: Johns Hopkins University Press, 2006.

Briggs Report on Nursing (1972) Available online at: https://navigator.health.org.uk/content/1972-briggs-committee-report-nursing-was-published (accessed on 23rd October 2019).

Buka P, 2nd ed. Patients Rights, Law and Ethics for Nurses, Boca Raton, CRC Press, 2015.

Declaration of Geneva (September 1948) Adopted by the General Assembly of World Medical Association at Geneva Switzerland. Available online at: http://www.cirp.org/library/ethics/geneva/ (Revised 6th June 2002).

Famous Trials. Available online at: https://www.famous-trials.com/nuremberg/1903-doctortrial (accessed on 19th July 2019).

Freegard H. ed. *Ethical practice for health professionals*. Melbourne: Thomson Learning, 2007.

Gillon R. Medical ethics: Four principles plus attention to scope. *BMJ* 1994; 309: 184–8.

Hippocratic Oath. *Translated by Michael North, National Library of Medicine*, 2002. Available online at: https://www.nlm.nih.gov/hmd/greek/greek_oath.html (accessed on 20th June 2019).

Holland S, ed. *Introducing nursing ethics: Themes in theory and practice*. Salisbury: APS, 2004.

Holocaust Encyclopedia. Available online at: https://encyclopedia.ushmm.org/content/en/article/nazi-medical-experiments (accessed on 29th July 2019).

International Council for Nurses. Available online on: https://www.icn.ch/ (accessed on 20th July 2019).

Managed Caremag. Available online at: https://www.managedcaremag.com/archives/1997/5/hammurabis-managed-health-care-circa-1700-bc (accessed on 20th July 2019).

NHS Constitution (2015) Available online at: https://www.gov.uk/government/publications/the-nhs-constitution-for-england (accessed on 22nd June 2019).

Nightingale F. *Nightingale notes on hospitals*, 3rd ed. Preface. Mineola, NY: Dover publications, 1863.

GMC guidance: Good practice in research and consent to research. Available online at: http://www.gmc-uk.org/static/documents/content/Good_practice_in_research_and_consent_to_research.pdf (accessed on 22nd June 2019).

Nuremberg Code. *Trials of war criminals before the Nuremberg Military Tribunals under Control Council Law No. 10*, Vol. 2, pp. 181–2. Washington: U.S. Government Printing Office, 1949.

Nursing and Midwifery Order (2001) Available online at: https://publications.parliament.uk/pa/ld200304/ldselect/ldconst/68/68we53.htmernment (accessed on 21st June 2019).

Publications Parliament. Available online at: https://publications.parliament.uk/pa/ld200304/ldselect/ldconst/68/68we53.htmernment (accessed on 22nd July 2019).

Report of the Morecambe Bay Investigation (2015) Available online at: https://assets.publishing.service.gov.uk/government/uploads/system/uploads/attachment_data/file/408480/47487_MBI_Accessible_v0.1.pdf (accessed on 21st June 2019).

Seedhouse D. *Ethics: The heart of health care*, 2nd ed. London: John Wiley & Sons, 1998.

Seedhouse D. *Values-based decision-making for the caring professions*. London: John Wiley & Son, 2009.

The Code (2018) Professional standards of practice and behaviour for nurses, midwives and nursing associates. Available online at: https://www.nmc.org.uk/standards/code/ (accessed on 19th July 2019).

Third Dynasty (Egypt, 2700 BCE) Available online at: http://www.levity.com/alchemy/islam22.html (accessed on 19th July 2019).

Human rights, the law

Chapter outline

Introduction

This chapter is concerned with basic human rights. These are fundamental to many legal principles. This chapter also establishes the link or marriage between ethics and law. The law of the land in any given country aims to establish order, social cohesion and regulation of human conduct. The law has developed from many sources, and these will be explored. Established legal frameworks have developed over time and will continue to evolve. Together with ethical principles, they are linked to relevant aspects of the law, with application to health care throughout the book. During the process of clinical decision-making, it is possible to consider both ethics and legal principles. There may, however, be a conflict between ethics and law as disciplines. Other cultural, societal, social or religious norms may also come into conflict with the law. The concept 'law' or 'legal' applies to a system of rules which set standards of conduct and which are applicable to a group or groups of people. The law defines people's rights and obligations. For a law to be effective, it should be enforceable, with consequences for failure to comply. One important element is that laws are derived from an authoritative source which give them efficacy. Like ethics, law evolves in response to the needs of a given society or country.

There are many branches of law. One common classification is *public law* which is within the public domain and *private law* which has been developed for the benefit of the private individual. Examples of public law are criminal law, administrative law and health and safety law. The private law includes examples such as family law, law of trusts and law of torts/delict which include negligence.

This chapter will focus on the law of tort, and it defines the duty of care and links this with clinical negligence. The NHS has set aside £65 billion in negligence (claim. org.uk). Other relevant branches of law will be addressed in the following chapters.

Sources of law

For most people, their first experience of 'laws' or 'regulation' may relate to rudimentary 'rules' experienced during their early developmental stages either at home or school. They may have experienced a dichotomy of 'dos' or 'don'ts'. Hopefully fundamental rules will have instilled in them, a 'sense moral' purpose and the ability to distinguish what is right from wrong or at least what is acceptable from what is not. This is a capacity for making decisions based on rational choice. The basis of compliance may be love or respect for parents/teachers. On the other hand, it could be argued that people have rational choice. They may adopt a different set of moral values and a way of life which may be shaped by peer pressure or society different to the one they were brought up in.

What is difficult to fathom is how it is possible within a given family, that some may deviate from expected norms of behaviour and go on to breach 'rules' which others may consider as sacrosanct. Personal experience is relevant for the beginnings of development of morals or moral values and respect for the law. It has been argued that accepting peers as equals is subject to the law as entitled individuals are entitled to protection under the law (Harris, 1985). When moral rules are breached, however, there are implications for potential abuses of human rights based on law and morality. State rules may be reprehensive (Wacks, 2017).

Albert Dicey (1835–1922), a classical jurist and legal philosopher, contributed to the debate on objectives of the law and its impact (in regulating human conduct). He held that society gives the law its pre-eminence over other disciplines such as natural law and ethics. He promoted parliamentary sovereignty. The UK Parliament has the right to make or unmake any laws it likes, hitherto, subject to the EU legislation. This means that no person is above the law, Tomkins and Turpin (2007) and central to their belief is the suggestion that for it to work, there is a need for the law to be impartial. Their central argument was that this would protect the human rights of citizens. Aspects of law, such as criminal law, employment law, contract and the law of torts, however, are founded on human rights and ethical principles, such as Principlism, the four principles:

> It would not be correct to say that every moral obligation involves a legal duty; but every legal duty is founded on a moral obligation. A legal common law duty is nothing else than the enforcing by law of that which is a moral obligation without legal enforcement.
>
> (Lord Chief Justice Coleridge, CJ at 453, R v Instan [1893] 1 QB at 453)

In the same vein, it is notable that, breach of ethical principles does not necessarily have a legal implication. From a nursing perspective, ethical beliefs of an individual nurse may influence their conduct on issues such as compassion and empathy toward their patients and how they should treat them with dignity and respect. When ethical dilemmas arise in healthcare decisions, nurses and healthcare professionals must follow the dictates of the law. Individual ethics are insufficient as the law takes precedence and establishes systems of governance in order to prevent chaos in a given society.

Without a universal definition, it is difficult to have clarity on the concept of law. This is not helped by the fact that in both Parliament (as a law-making body) and the courts conflict may arise as the judges struggle to match the intention of Parliament with preceding case law. For most people the meaning of 'legal concepts' may be shrouded in mystery and be open to subjective interpretations and argument during this process called statutory interpretation. Others, Aquinas (1225–74) in Summa Theologiae in McDermitt (1997), held that individuals have a free will to choose to follow or adopt as their own individual standards of morality. People develop a 'moral fibre' based on religion, culture upbringing and education or individual experience. There will be other variables, highlighting similarities as well as differences, depending on local, national or international values. There is a need for asserting order and harmony. This should be the role of the state, through all its three arms: the legislature (Parliament), the executive (government) and the judiciary (courts). The last branch acts as guardian of the rule of law by interpreting the will of Parliament as well as developing the principles of case law. The study of morality otherwise known as moral philosophy or ethics is concerned with right and wrong of human actions.

Professional ethical or moral values inevitably underpin practice in some cases, and subject to the law. Established ethical frameworks are respected by most healthcare professionals and may influence dealing with ethical dilemmas arising during the delivery of care. Ethical principles, however, do not have the force of law.

> Ethics is about moral choices. It is about the values that lie behind them, the reasons people give for them … it is about innocence and guilt, right and wrong and what it means to live a good or bad life … dilemmas of life, death …
>
> (Thompson, 2003)

Ethics is 'the rational discussion of that process' (decision-making) (Thompson, 2003, p. 1). Ethics may be called upon when faced with a dilemma, and professionals should first look to their own code of conduct for guidance. Clinical judgements may also be influenced by the individual professional's ethical beliefs based on their cultural and/or religious background.

> Whether a society has an ethical system can be recognised by it having a mental construct of values which are expressed as principles to be invoked and interpreted in guiding social behaviour (i.e. that which has meaning for others) and in judging it in gradations of good or bad.
>
> (Singer, 2003, p. 17)

Moral dilemmas may arise when clinical decisions are made. The role of ethics is limited as the law supersedes any decision-making. There are exceptions to the rule, which allow for conscientious objection based on moral or other grounds.

Conscientious objection and the law

What happens when a clinician has a conscientious objection to participating in a medical procedure? Ethical principles underpin the law (this may also coincide with individual or professional values). They may therefore interpret the law based on their personal ethical, customary or religious values. The tension between law and ethics will be highlighted throughout.

There are two exceptions in law. A nurse who is a conscientious objector may re-sort to their 'conscience' for guidance or may indeed be exempt from participating in certain procedures. When an ethical dilemma arises, there may be considerations conflicting with the legal principles; nevertheless, the law should always prevail over ethics. It is therefore possible that may be scope for some exceptions to this general rule. The two examples are conscientious objection under the Abortion Act 1967 and the Human Fertilisation and Embryology Act 1991:

> 4. Conscientious objection to participation in treatment.
> (1) Subject to subsection (2) of this section, no person shall be under any duty, whether by contract or by any statutory or other legal requirement, to participate in any treatment authorised by this Act to which he has a conscientious objection:
>
> > Provided that in any legal proceedings the burden of proof of conscientious objection shall rest on the person claiming to rely on it.
> >   (Section 4 (1) Abortion Act 1967)

A doctor also has the right to conscientious objection, but they are expected to provide the patient with objective and non-judgemental advice on treatment (Paragraph 52 of the GMC's Good Medical Practice, 2018).

Box 2.1 Case: Greater Glasgow Health Board v Doogan & Anor [2014] UKSC 68

Morals and conscientious objection

This case was initiated by a senior nurse (band 7) midwife (supervising junior midwives) who sought clarification on whether conscientious objection on religious grounds in-cluded 'the entitlement to refuse to delegate, supervise and/or support staff in the par-ticipation in and provision of care to patients undergoing termination of pregnancy or feticide throughout the termination process'.

Held: This right did not extend to conscientious objection for staff supervising staff who are participating in terminations of pregnancy.

Abortion Act 1967 is currently not applicable to Northern Ireland.

The other exception is provided under the Human Fertilisation and Embryology Act 1990.

> 38 Conscientious objections
> (1) No person who has a conscientious objection to participating in any activity governed by this Act shall be under any duty, however arising, to do so.
> (2) In any legal proceedings the burden of proof of conscientious objection shall rest on the person claiming to rely on it.

In respect of Section 38 (2) above, the burden of proof rests with the conscientious objector; however, this is different in Scotland where it is enough for the conscientious objector to swear an oath to this effect.

Sources impacting on law

Ethics is one key source of law which is intertwined with it but can also be at variance. Other sources of the law include international treaties (as well as the European legislation) such as the International Declaration on Human Rights 1948. Other main sources are national legislation, which consists of statutes or acts of parliament, and delegated legislation, which is laws from government departments, local authorities regulated professional bodies empowered by parliament to legislate. Examples are regulatory authorities such as the Department of Health and Social Care, with devolved departments in Scotland, Wales and Northern Ireland.

The Roman invasion of Western Europe meant that Latin terminology is still dominant in legal principles and use of terminology today. In contrast to English common law, Scots law developed its own unique systems, such as the law of delict as well as influences from a number of sources. There are some principles rooted in the Roman-Dutch law traditions (which affected Scots law through trading links and scholars studying law in Holland and France, through links with the Kirk (Church) in the seventeenth and eighteenth centuries). Notable is the part French law played, following the signing of the 'Auld Alliance' between John Balliol of Scotland and Philip IV of France (1295) against Edward I of England. With Scottish jurists travelling across the sea this meant the inevitable influence of French law with '... dual citizenship in both countries (which) was eventually revoked by the French government in 1903' (Historic UK, https://www.historic-uk.com/HistoryUK/HistoryofScotland/The-Auld-Alliance-France-Scotland/).

In comparison, English private law has stronger routes in the feudal system, with the influence of the church in both traditions in areas such as family, succession and property laws. Institutional writers like Professor Erskine's Institutes (1730) and Viscount Stair's Institution (1773) also provided a unique source for Scotland and are often quoted as authority in Scots law (Nicolson and Erskine, 1871). The Union of Crowns (1603) influenced both countries, with more similarities between the two systems, though nevertheless distinct principles in some areas.

Following the 1707 Union of Parliaments, the House of Lords became the final court of appeal for all cases including Scottish cases, with the result that English law could be applied to Scottish cases and vice versa. In criminal law, however, appeals continue to he heard under the Scottish High Court of Justiciary (criminal appeal court) sitting as the final court.

The main classifications of sources are primary and secondary.

Primary sources of law are international treaties, the European Parliament and the UK Parliament and assemblies (pertaining to their respective laws). These are in the form of statute law.

Secondary sources originate from multiple sources. Unlike countries like France, with the bulk of the law being codified, UK laws have developed from a variety of sources.

Delegated legislation empowers local authorities and government departments to pass delegated legislation. This is supplementary legislation which is enabled by a parent statute or act of parliament from which it is derived. Additionally, by-laws are from professional bodies established by royal charter, such as the nursing and Midwifery

Council (NMC). Another important source is common law, when the courts develop principles of law based on previous decisions of the same or higher court.

Up to until Brexit, the European Parliament has had authority to legislate for UK law – by accession and membership of the European Union under the (now repealed) Communities Act 1962 (Blair, 2010). There are four main political institutions of the European Union (EU):

- *Council of Ministers*: This is composed of representative ministers from each member state. This is the most effective group as the law-making body of the EU.
- *Commission*: This is the administrative arm of the EU and is composed of technocrats and administrators who are responsible for drafting legislation. This is the equivalent of the civil service with the function of supporting the Council of Ministers. It is headed by an unelected president.
- *Assembly* (the European Parliament): Unlike the UK Parliament, this body has no law-making powers. Its main function is to debate on topics of interest to the EU, which may be contemporary to and of interest to Europe. Its consensus-based recommendations will be the basis for recommendations or guidelines for ministers on the Council of Ministers when legislating. They may also influence governments as they relay decisions to influence their own national parliaments. The assembly is also responsible for electing officials such as judges.

European Court of Justice is the highest court in the EU, which should not be confused with the European Court of Human Rights. Sometimes known as the Court of Justice of the European Communities, it is based in Luxembourg. Each EU state has a sovereign jurisdiction of its different legal systems. This court is responsible for adjudicating between the EU and member states or in an interstate dispute on the interpretation of European law.

For example:

a. between the European Commission and a member state which fails to implement a European Union directive,
b. between the European Commission and a member state, claiming that the European Commission has acted ultra vires, outside its jurisdiction,
c. between national courts from member states asking for clarification on the validity of specific EC legislation (subject to Article 189/EC, which defines the method extent and application of the European laws). This will change with Brexit.

Judges, representing member states, normally serve for a renewable term of six years.

The European Court of Human Rights in Strasbourg was established for addressing human rights, currently under the European Convention on Human Rights 1950. Cases may be launched on an appeal basis or may go directly to this court.

There are three classifications of EU laws:

Regulations, which are binding to member states, must be applied directly in their entirety.
Directives serve as mechanisms for bringing into line national laws, subject to an agreed timetable for the implementation. An example is the EU Data Protection Directive 1995, which had as its main aim protection of personal information and harmonization of privacy laws within the EU. In the UK, the result was the

Data Protection Act 1998 on privacy and the General Data Protection Regulation (GDPR) 2018 for better protection of individual data.

Decisions are the legal decisions (or case law) of the European Court of Justice. This effectively modifies the basic constitutional principle on Parliamentary Sovereignty which means that it (parliament) can make or unmake any laws based on a majority vote.

European laws are equally binding and applicable to all countries of the UK. The law can be changed by the UK Parliament subject to the EU European Court of Justice's interpretation. Professional bodies such as the Nursing and Midwifery Council (NMC) are a source of delegated legislation which regulates professional conduct. Another important source of law is case law. The authority of case laws is based on 'judicial precedent', or *stare decisis* (Latin), meaning 'to stand by matters decided'. A decision binds a court of a lower level decision of a lower court. This doctrine defines strict 'following [of] legal rules' or principles as laid down in previous judicial decisions unless they contravene the ordinary principles of justice. This means that a court decision is bound by a previous decision of a higher court. This may present difficulties as miscarriages of justice and grounds for appeal result.

In jurisprudence, legal principles may be the basis of arguments resulting in legal disputes, and challenges to a superior court. Statutory Interpretation of the law depends on the judges' 'human' understanding and application, hence the individual judge's interpretation of the law may be influenced by their own ethical values. The interpretation of the intent of parliament 'Statutory Interpretation' means that the intent of parliament and application of the law may be disputed, hence the reason for appealing to a higher court, as the court may get it wrong.

This may change post-Brexit. The European Withdrawal Act 2018 repealed the Communities Act 1972 (above) which admitted the UK to the EU. The effect will be;

1. Retaining most of the existing EU law as UK domestic law after Brexit in order to ensure the continuity and completeness of the UK's legal system.
2. Parliament will have wide powers to amend that retained EU law to reflect the changed status of the UK after Brexit while mitigating any problems caused by exiting from the EU.

Emerging human rights and the law

From an international perspective, human rights were more focussed post-Second World War, when a United Nations-sponsored International Treaty emerged as the Universal Declaration of Human Rights 1948, with 30 articles. This was adopted by several countries which adopted this and specific articles on human rights. The Universal Declaration subsequently became a United Nations the General Assembly Resolution 217 on 10 December 1948 in Paris. European Convention on Human Rights (ECHR) 1950.

The UK is a signatory to this international human rights legislation and provides for human rights through the Human Rights Act 1998. The UK now must subscribe to the (ECHR) 1950 the Human Rights Act (HRA) 1998 which give the UK courts power to implement it. Alternative cases may be heard on appeal to the European Court of Human Rights. There are 17 articles in total, and only relevant ones will be considered below.

The general categories of rights under the HRA (1998) are classified as follows (Ministry of Justice, 2006):

- unqualified/absolute rights, which cannot be amended – Articles 2, 3, 4(1) and 7;
- qualified rights, which may be modified by the state in extreme circumstances, e.g. in a state of emergency – Articles 4(2), 5, 6 and 12;
- limited rights, which are subject to limitation by the state depending on a given society's needs – Articles 8, 10 and 11.

Relevant aspects of the articles affect the way we care for patients. Since 2 October 2000, public bodies and local authorities now have a duty to safeguard individual rights and these can be enforced in UK courts (Makkan, 2000). Judges have the power to refer to Parliament for clarification of the intention of legislature, if the law is uncertain. Some of the aspects of the Human Rights Act Schedule affecting patient care are as follows:

Article 2 – Right to life. Everyone's right to life shall be protected by law. No one shall be deprived of his life intentionally save in the execution of a sentence of a court following his conviction of a crime for which this penalty is provided by law.

This places basic human rights at the centre of governing and protecting citizens from arbitrary actions by other, more powerful citizens who may choose to usurp their rights. This was central to a framework for human rights to which signatories signed up. The UK enacted the Human Rights Act 1998 which received royal assent on 9 November 1998, 25 years after Britain became a signatory of the then European Economic Community (EEC), on 1 January 1973. The most important principle embodied in this piece of legislation (Leckie and Pickergill, 2000) is that 'everyone's right to life shall be protected by the law' (Article 2, European Convention on the Protection of Human Rights and Fundamental Freedoms 1950). The European convention may be used to apply human rights, by state versus state or individual versus state, in the European Court of Human Rights (De Than and Shorts, 2013).

Article 3 – Prohibition of torture. None shall be subjected to torture or inhuman or degrading treatment or punishment. An example of an alleged breach of this article is illustrated in the following case:

Box 2.2 Case: NHS Trust A v M and NHS Trust B v H [2001] Fam 348

A hospital sought permission to discontinue artificial hydration and nutrition to a patient who in 1997 had been diagnosed as being in a 'permanent vegetative state'. The court held that Article 2 imposed a positive obligation to give treatment where that is in the best interests of the patient – but not where it would be futile. Discontinuing treatment would not be an intentional deprivation of life under Article 2, and provided that withdrawing treatment was in line with a respected body of medical opinion, and that the patient would be unaware of the treatment and not suffering, there would be no torture under Article 3.

Article 5 – Deprivation of Liberty Safeguarding (DoLS) now called Liberty Protection Safeguards (LPS) since 2018. This includes imprisonment and is applicable to limiting a vulnerable person's freedom.

Article 8 – Right to respect for private and family life. Everyone has the right to his private and family life, his home and his correspondence. There shall be no interference by a public authority with the exercise of this right except such as is in accordance with the law. This is consistent with the patient's right of autonomy, consent to treatment and informed choice.

Article 14 – Requires that all the rights and freedoms set out in the Act must be protected and applied without discrimination. This outlaws discrimination. Under the Equality Act 2010, this may also be on various grounds such as age, gender and sexuality.

Article 17 – Prohibition of abuse of rights. Nothing in this convention may be interpreted as implying for any state, group or person any right to engage in any activity or perform any act aimed at the destruction of any of the rights and freedoms set forth herein or at their limitation than is provided for in the convention.

The Human Rights Act 1998 (HRA) enabled the European Convention on Human Rights 1950. This requires UK courts to interpret the law in compatibility with this statute. UK courts also have a duty to refer the matter to Parliament if there is conflict with existing legislation, thus enabling them to make a 'declaration of incompatibility' and apply to UK legislation, even if this is in breach of European legislation (Welch, in Addis and Morrow, 2005). The onus is on Parliament to decide on amending the existing legislation in question, to bring it into line with European legislation. A claimant may appeal or take their case directly to the European Court of Human Rights (ECHR) in Strasbourg. The extent of the human rights applies to public bodies only and does not cover private organizations. While patient A, in an NHS trust hospital, may be able to complain based on the HRA 1998 Act, patient B in a private hospital would not be entitled to do so. The statute also covers those in employment who may wish to litigate against an employer. Thus, the act creates both civil and criminal rights. Membership of the EU has made it possible for the 17 rights outlined in the Human Rights Act schedule to be enforceable in UK courts normally within three months if this is for a declaration of rights only. If, however, a complainant is seeking damages for breach of human rights, they must file the case within a year of the date of the alleged incident. However, a patient going to litigation should be aware that the time limit for litigation under the HRA varies depending on the brief (the document stating the facts and points of law of a client's case). Respect for Patients' human rights should be fundamental in nursing RCN (2012).

UK courts may in the first instance make a declaration of human rights and award damages, if infringement of human rights has been proven, or opt to make a declaration only if they feel that damages are not warranted. For any cases which do not fall within the provisions of the HRA 1998 Act, the court will apply existing domestic law.

Subject to the Limitation Act 1980 and the Prescription and Limitation (Scotland) Act 1973, a litigant seeking redress normally has a three-year limitation, at the discretion of the courts.

Duty of care, and standard of care

Box 2.3 Thinking point

Reflecting on your professional duty of care.

One day while taking a short walk to your workplace, you come across a head-on collision, about 200 metres outside the hospital.

Both drivers seem to be fine but in shock. One of the drivers is a young woman in her early thirties who is screaming and distraught, saying her 78-year-old mother stumbled and collapsed as she tried to get out of the car. She is not breathing.

1   What is your duty of care towards the passenger and these other road users?
2   Consider patients who are within your remit of care; how do their rights fit in with the duty of care?
3   What ethical principles are related to the duty of care?

The 'duty of care' principle has evolved from a moral sense of responsibility or obligation. The difference is that apart from social isolation, ethics alone may not be enough to enforce the duty of care or to impose sanctions for breach. The term 'duty of care' has developed with a moral influence it. It is the basis of human obligations toward others who may be affected by our actions (Elliot and Quinn, 2009). This is easier to establish where there is a relationship which is fiduciary and based on trust.

Box 2.4 Thinking point

Joe, a 40-year-old man with learning disabilities, is admitted to A&E with pneumonia. He is normally independent and self-caring, receiving minimum support in a warden-controlled accommodation. He becomes aggressive and slaps the male nurse who was admitting him as he was hurting him with a needle. The SHO is angry and threatens to refuse treating him. During an altercation, Joe discharges himself but shortly after collapses in the hospital grounds on his way to the bus stop and had to be readmitted in a very unstable and life-threatening condition.

1   What was the hospital's duty of care towards Joe?
2   How should the staff proceed?

The following landmark House of Lords case originating in Scotland defined the duty of care while establishing the 'neighbour principle'. This is still good law today in the UK as well as being consistently applied to clinical negligence cases in other common law systems worldwide. The principle of 'duty of care' became law when the ethical basis was borrowed and defined on the landmark case of Donoghue v Stevenson [1932] AC 562 HL. Famously dubbed as the 'case of the snail and the ginger beer bottle', where a customer had consumed remains of a decomposed snail and then successfully claimed for negligence in tort.

> **Box 2.5 Case: Donoghue v Stevenson HL [1932] HL All ER Rep1**
>
> The claimant visited a café with a friend, who had bought her ice cream and a drink of ginger beer. The café owner poured some of the drink over her ice cream, and she consumed it. When she poured the rest of it, she found the decomposing remains of a dead snail. The claimant became unwell as a result. She could, however, not claim against the manufacturer in contract law as she had no contract with him.
>
> Held: The claim for damages for negligence (in tort) against the manufacturer was entitled to succeed despite not having contractual right.

The following dicta are usually accepted as a definition in the corner stone of tort law (delict in Scotland), and more specifically applicable to clinical negligence:

> You must take reasonable care to avoid acts or omissions which you can reasonably foresee would be likely to injure your neighbour.

The principle that a manufacturer who allows a defective product to leave their possession for distribution for sale owes a duty of care to their ultimate consumer is now applicable to a healthcare relationship;

> In response to the question 'who is my neighbour?'... 'persons who are so closely affected by my act that I ought reasonably to have them in my contemplation as being affected when I am directing my mind to the acts or omissions which are called in question'.
>
> (Lord Atkins, at p. 580, Donoghue v Stevenson [1932]).

This means that a duty of care will arise when there is an allegation of negligence, and where care is said to have fallen below certain specific standards. Based on this principle and the fiduciary relationship (based on trust) there is little difficulty for the courts to establish that a healthcare professional who is responsible for treating a patient owes them a duty of care. This duty is not to harm them as well as to avoid omissions, which may cause them (patients) harm (Mason et al., 2010). This principle can be applied to any trusting relationship between teacher and child, driver instructor and learner driver. This duty of care also applies to a variety of such contractual relationships between parties such as pilot and passengers, tradesperson and customer.

The tort of negligence requires healthcare professionals, in response to a claim for clinical negligence to be able to justify their decisions and actions. This will be judged in comparison to the standards of their peers, the Bolam Test. This is where evidence-based practice is applicable in defence of negligence claims.

The law of tort or delict (Scotland), which deals with claims in damages for personal injury, has prerequisites to be met before a victim of clinical negligence can successfully raise a claim for damages in court. They are called 'hurdles' which need to overcome before negligence is established in Donoghue v Stevenson (1932).

The plaintiff or victim is owed a duty of care by the defendant or defender (Scotland). This is to prevent unwarranted and frivolous claims to limit the claims. The nurse owes duty of care to all within their remit of care. An 'off-duty' nurse's duty of care is not expected to demonstrate skills beyond a reasonable response: for example,

Basic Life Support skills and not 'miracles' and specialist skills without a suitable environment and support.

- The plaintiff must have proof of breach of that duty by the defendant. There must be enough proximity in their relationship. This could be the most difficult aspect to prove as this is relative.
- Establish that the plaintiff suffered harm as a result of the alleged breach of the duty of care.
- Did the alleged breach cause the harm in question, *a causal nexus*? There must be a chain of causation or a close connection of the actions of the defendant?

In the mind of a defendant or defender (Scotland), there should be reasonable foreseeability (or as common sense predicts), and this also pertains to the limitation of damages. This is a matter in the public interest to limit frivolous claims and prevent floodgates. The law provides for the right of the defendant to be heard and counter-argue their case (Hodgson and Lewthwaite, 2004). One example is a response that a victim caused or contributed to their own injury and were therefore negligent. Where this is proven the court may award damages on a quantum basis. This means that this is proportionate to their contribution.

The duty of care is developed further when standards of care may be called in question. The following case was important for healthcare professionals responding to allegations of negligence.

Box 2.6 Case: Bolam v Friern Hospital Management Committee [1957] 1 WLR 582, the court

This reinforces the importance of following evidence-based practice, Lord McNair's judgement, regarding a patient at a Friern Hospital Management Committee hospital. He agreed to undergo electro-convulsive therapy without having any muscle relaxant. His body was not restrained during the procedure. He suffered serious injuries, including fractures of the acetabula. He sued the Committee for compensation for negligence, arguing that defendants were negligent for:

1 not administering relaxants,
2 not restraining him,
3 not warning him about the risks involved.

Argued that the defendants owed him a duty of care.

It was held that

> ... he (or she) (a doctor or healthcare professional) is not guilty of negligence if he (or she) has acted in accordance with a practice accepted as proper by a responsible body of medical men (or women) skilled in that particular art ... I do not think there is much difference in sense. It is just a different way of expressing the same thought. Putting it the other way around, a man is not negligent, if he is acting in accordance with such a practice, merely because there is a body of opinion who would take a contrary view.
> (McNair J. in, Bolam v Friern Hospital Management Committee [1957] 1 WLR 582)

A plea entered by the hospital in defence, based on the Bolam Test failed in the subsequent case:

Box 2.7 Case: Wilsher v Essex Area Health Authority (1987) QB 730.CA, 1988 AC 1074

The Claimant was born Prematurely. Subsequently the Defendant negligently gave the Claimant excess oxygen. A catheter was wrongly inserted into his vein on two occasions instead of his artery and as a result, he developed an incurable eye condition. The court accepted that although his blindness could have been caused by one of any other conditions found in Premature babies. The hospital admitted only negligence in genera/on that basis. The court upheld the objective standard in respect of a junior doctor who could not argue his <u>inexperience</u> as a reason to avoid liability. The hospital was found to be liable.

The interpretation of the Bolam Test was re-affirmed applied in the Appeal Court where the House of Lords held that this was insufficient on its own but must be supported by evidence-based practice, *Bolitho v City & Hackney Health Authority [1997] 3 WLR 1151*. A significant decision on the Bolam Test was Lord Scarman's approach in the following case:

Box 2.8 Case: Sidaway v. Bethlem Royal Hospital and Ors. [1985] AC 871; [1985] 1 All ER 643

Sidaway brought an action in negligence against Bethlem Royal Hospital and the hospital's surgeon after she was left severely disabled from a spinal operation. Ms Sidaway, who suffered from constant shoulder and neck pains, was advised by a surgeon employed by the hospital to have an operation on her spinal column to relieve her pain. The surgeon had warned her of the inherent risks of the operation but allegedly failed to warn her of the risk of spinal damage which could lead to partial paralysis. The risk of such damage was estimated at less than 1 per cent and would be present even if the operation was performed with due care and skill. The risk materialized during Ms Sidaway's operation and left her severely disabled after the operation. She brought an action against the hospital and the surgeon's estate (since he had died before the matter could go to trial), claiming damages for personal injury. As the surgical procedure had been performed accurately, Ms Sidaway based her case on the surgeon's failure to inform her of all the risks of the operation.

https://www.globalhealthrights.org/pdf.php?ID=1173

Montgomery v Lanarkshire Health Board [2015] UKSC 11, overruled the above case and considered that a defence for clinical negligence as linked to information-giving in order to obtain consent. Adopting Lord Scarman's (dissenting) minority approach that, the law should recognize the right of a patient with capacity to be informed about material risks, except in emergencies and where a person lacks capacity. The Bolam Test is still relevant, but this does not apply to consent cases.

Litigation and Compensation

The basic principle behind the right to compensation of a victim is based on fairness and the unequal relationship between perpetrator and victim. The duty of case may be applied from a broader perspective, in a fiduciary relationship. The law may be invoked not only to define rights and create obligations but also to define sanctions against those who may fail to comply with its dictates; the link between ethics and law is easy to see. Accountability or liability lies at the heart of litigation. The duty of care is not difficult to prove where there is a relationship based on trust and an unequal balance of power and control. This was highlighted in the following unusual case:

Box 2.9 Case: R v Instan [1893] 1 QB at 453

D. lived with her aunt, who developed gangrene in her leg and became totally dependent and unable to call for help. The defendant failed to feed her aunt or to call for medical help, even though she (the defendant) remained in the house and continued to eat her aunt's food. The aunt's dead body was found in the house decomposing for about a week.

Held: The defendant had a duty of care to supply her deceased aunt with enough food to maintain life. In addition, the death of her aunt had been accelerated due to her neglect of this duty of care.

The law should be accessible to all citizens in its application and key characteristics of the law must have certainty with an identity or an ability to test this:

- it should be impersonal and apply either to all citizens or to a specified group of people; the law has an ability to create some rights while defining corresponding obligations and this include the right of an injured party to seek compensation.

The development of law of obligations can be traced back to ancient societies' attempt to establish some order. One dated example is that of ancient codification of law by Hammurabi (ca. 1792–50 BC), of Mesopotamia; Hammurabi's Code was a systematic code of laws (with 282 articles in total). The aim of the code was to regulate human conduct, both in private and in public; nevertheless, this was mostly meting out justice on an 'eye for an eye' basis. The following aspects of the Hammurabi Code are examples of the application of this principle:

218. If a physician make a large incision with the operating knife, and kill him, or open a tumour with the operating knife, and cut out the eye, his hands shall be cut off ….
221. If a physician heals the broken bone or diseased soft part of a man, the patient shall pay the physician five shekels in money ….
229. If a builder build a house for someone, and does not construct it properly, and the house which he built fall in and kill its owner, then that builder shall be put to death.

(https://hekint.org/2017/01/30/oaths-codes-and-charters-in-medicine-over-the-ages/)

As laws developed in democratic western societies, there have been recognized channels for individuals to seek redress and/or to assert their rights. The aim of litigation is to seek damages in compensation (or reparation) for the harm (or personal injury) they (victim) may have suffered as a result of the wrongdoer's (defendant, or defender in Scots law) negligent actions or omissions. The aim of tort law or delict (Scots law) is to make reparation or restitution (Scots law) for any harm done. A patient who suffers harm as result of a healthcare professional's negligence is entitled to damages in compensation for personal injury. The main hurdle for the litigant is proving the causation by the defendant. 'Quantum' or 'quantification' is a measure of damages. Several categories may be included, with the main ones in tort being classed under the headings of general speculative or special damages. Occasionally, exemplary (punitive) damages may be awarded, for example, in cases where the courts feel the importance of making a public statement, in order to prevent something from happening again. Such damages are not normally awardable to victims.

General damages: 'If the victim sought a money award for pain and suffering, mental anguish, and loss of consortium *(association)*, these would be classified as general damages' (Free Dictionary, accessed 2013). Examples of headings for the injury the claimant received are pain, loss and suffering, and loss of amenity.

Special damages: They are compensatory, called *restitutio in integrum* in Latin, meaning aiming to return persons to the position they would have been in, had they not endured the alleged injury. For example, if a person was negligently injured in a surgical operation, 'the victim could seek damages that could cover medical expenses … and the loss of earnings now and in the future' (Free Dictionary, accessed 2013). This would also include nursing home care and adaptations to living accommodation.

What are reasons why people sue for damages or compensation? The main reasons for compensation may be as follows:

- Pain and suffering, mainly physical but also associated psychological harm is admissible.
- Costs for ongoing treatment as a direct result of the harm
- Compensation for loss of function, activities or hobbies
- Loss of current and future earnings
- The cost of any extra care or equipment which the victim may need
- The cost of adapting home

It is therefore important for healthcare staff to be aware of patients' rights and how to safeguard these patients. Laws may be subject to review as time moves on, in any given society or within a group of people with a common interest. While most laws are promulgated by democratically elected government, in theocratic governments laws may nevertheless be imposed from a superior order, such as the theocratic or the dictate of an autocratic ruler, as they deem fit. In a theocracy, which claims a divine right, there are those who may learn to give laws their pre-eminence in the belief that all laws come from a divine source, through a theocratic authority. As a representative of (theocratic) authority, some rulers may abuse their subjects' rights. Acceptable forms of authority in a democracy emanate from elected representatives. The judiciary should be an arm of the government for safeguarding and defining the rights of citizens. In comparison, most people would also accept that in the scientific world there are accepted laws of nature which if breached may have disastrous consequences.

Davies (1998) acknowledges that there may be difficulties in accessing evidence which is mainly in medical records. The reality of the matter is that over many years, witnesses may move, forget what happened or die before the case comes to court. Delays may work against the claimant. The Access to Health Records Act 1990, gives a patient or their representative a right to access non computerized clinical records, with the Data Protection Act 1998 regulating computerized ones.

Box 2.10 Case: Johnson v Fourie [2011] EWHC 1062 (QB)

A patient underwent cosmetic surgery then suffered from severe disfigurement and disablement due to the surgeon's negligent action. The surgeon admitted liability.

Held: Negligence by the surgeon had been proven. The litigant was awarded damages of nearly £6 million.

Until the enactment of the Crown Proceedings Act (CPA) 1947, the crown or the government, as its representative, could not be sued. Following removal of crown immunity, it is now possible for the crown to have liability in tort/delict, with a government minister having nominal liability (Cracknell, 2004). In fact, to the present day, subject to Section 40(1) of the CPA 1947, the queen cannot be made personally liable in tort. Additionally, judges cannot be sued for action in the process of dispensing their duties.

With modern-day advancements in medicine, patients have also come to have raised expectations (Davies, 1998). In addition, due to current policy standards, any high expectations on the quality of care may be reinforced.

A victim claiming damages must also establish (on a balance of probabilities) the facts, which can be 'hurdles' in the progress before the courts can award damages for personal injury in tort (McHale and Tingle, 2007; Brazier and Mc Cave, 2014). In contrast, a criminal conviction requires to go beyond reasonable doubt. The most common claim in a personal injury case is for 'negligence' and the time limit for this is three years (Limitations Act 1980 or the Prescription and Limitation [Scotland] Act 1973). The effect is that court proceedings must be issued within three years of the victim first being aware of having suffered an injury. A victim claiming damages must establish the facts (on a balance of probabilities). They must pass the 'hurdles' before the courts can award damages for personal injury in tort (McHale and Tingle., 2007). Some claims fall short of the requirements at the initial hurdles as it can be difficult to prove clinical negligence at times especially where there are latent complications of a clinical event, which may surface a long time after. Latent claims may be allowed at the discretion of the court.

There are different time limits within which a victim must begin legal action in a personal injury claim. For deliberately caused personal injury, however, the limitation period is six years from the date of injury.

Some victims of clinical negligence may not bother to raise an action for personal injury, with only a relatively small proportion doing so. 76 per cent of these were unsuccessful (Mason et al., 2010). Latent claims may be allowed at the discretion of the court.

Litigation usually involves an uphill struggle and most victims cannot afford the hassle, time and money to fight a case. In order to recover damages, a claimant must establish on a balance of probabilities that the defendant's negligence had a material effect on the outcome of the disease. The burden of proof (on a balance of probabilities) lies with the victim.

For healthcare professionals who hold themselves out as having a specialist skill, they will be judged by the standards of a reasonably competent healthcare professional. The standard of care expected by the courts is that of the 'reasonable' clinician based on peers, which is the higher rather than the lower one, and the Bolam test, established in *Bolam v Friern Hospital Management Committee* [1957] 1 WLR 582.

Davies (1998) acknowledged potential difficulties in accessing evidence, which is mainly retained in clinical records. The Access to Health Records Act 1990 gives a patient or their representative a right to access non-computerized clinical records, with the Data Protection Act 1998 regulating computerized ones.

Nursing regulation and law

The NMC was established under the Nursing and Midwifery Order 2001 ('the order') and came into being on 1 April 2002. Before this, in 1983, the UK Central Council for Nursing, Midwifery and Health Visiting (UKCC) had been set up, with its main objective as one of maintaining a register of UK nurses, midwives and health visitors, as well as providing guidance to registrants; professional misconduct issues with national boards (with a remit for nurse education) were created for each of the UK countries.

With increased autonomous practice and accountability, the days of the nurse who was subservient to 'doctors' orders' are now behind us.

An individual nurse may, however, choose to act contrary to professional standards of ethics and standards or morality, *R v Allitt, 1992 [2007] EWHC 2845*, and they will be judged by the law as well as by 'accepted' societal norms due to the overlap. This may harm the patient in their care. The question posed is whether it is the norm for professionals to identify their own individual morality with 'professional ethics', which happens to be embodied in the law, in the form of the NMC Code (2018).

Nowadays, nurses function even more autonomously but, more importantly, collaboratively within a multi-disciplinary team setting. This collaboration includes the doctor, who is a key member of the team, with the patient at the centre of treatment. The concepts of scope of practice and accountability are such that it is inevitable for nurses to have more regulation in a climate of more awareness of patient rights in the face of increased litigation.

> Nursing encompasses autonomous and collaborative care of individuals of all ages, families, groups and communities, sick or well and in all settings. Nursing includes the promotion of health, prevention of illness, and the care of ill, disabled and dying people. Advocacy, promotion of a safe environment, research, participation in shaping health policy and in patient and health systems management, and education are also key nursing roles.
> (https://www.icn.ch/nursing-policy/nursing-definitions)

It was important that nurses are represented by professional nurses who regulate the profession, and this is applicable to professional bodies such as the Nursing and Midwifery Council (NMC). The NMC have legal authority through their Council which was created by royal charter to regulate standards of professional behaviour for nurses (Hinchcliff et al., 2008).

It is permissible, however, for nurses to appeal to the High Court against an NMC decision (in this case against being struck off).

Box 2.11 Case: Kituma v Nursing and Midwifery Council (Rev 1) [2009] EWHC 373 (Admin) (9 March 2009)

A midwife performed an episiotomy contrary to established procedure trust policy; it was held that due to the harm suffered by the patient and the failure to follow procedure trust policy by the appellant, the appeal was entitled to fail.

Conclusion

Understanding of a clear concept of law is necessary in clinical decision-making. Patients' rights should be at the centre of service provision. Nurses must be advocates for patients' basic human rights. The issue of patients' rights is fundamental to nurses' understanding of their clients' needs. The European Convention on Human Rights 1950 enabled by the Human Rights Act 1998 and related legislation were key in defining these rights. The full effect of human rights legislation has yet to be tested. For example, breach of the patient's right of choice may result in infringement of other statutory provisions with not only breach of human rights but also an indictable criminal offence but may also attract civil action and a lawsuit for damages for compensation for personal harm. Patients are now more questioning and aware of their rights than ever, and the threat of litigation is real. Should a patient ever become a victim of clinical negligence, the trust between them and healthcare professionals may be eroded. Where partnership and transparency are present, healthcare professionals should work together and in collaboration with the patient (NHS Constitution, 2019). Most patients are vulnerable, especially if they lack the mental capacity to assert their rights.

Human rights are open to abuse, by those purportedly representing or advocating for vulnerable people. What is needed in safeguarding is a balance between interests of patients, and those of other stakeholders, and those of healthcare professionals; the provisions of the law must be followed. Whatever clinical decision is made in respect of treatment must have the patient at the centre of decisions. There is still a possibility that occasionally, patients' rights may be eroded, by family members, patients' carers, healthcare professionals and/or the courts. The law aims to define those rights and to set the boundaries. Challenges may be present in some circumstances such as where people lack capacity or in emergency situations. Ethics should empower nurses and together with the law safeguard these patients' rights, not merely to remind nurses' 'consciences'. It is nevertheless for the law to define and regulate human rights.

References

Abortion Act 1967.

Access to Health Records Act 1990.

Addis M and Morrow P, eds. *Your rights: The liberty guide to human rights.* London: Liberty, 2005.

Blair A. *The European Union since 1945*, 2nd ed. Harlow: Person Education Limited, 2010.

Bolam v Friern Hospital Management Committee [1957] 1 WLR 582.

Bolitho v City & Hackney Health Authority [1997] 3 WLR 1151.

Brazier M and Mc Cave E. *Medicine, patients and the law*, 6th ed. Manchester: Manchester University Press, 2014.

Communities Act 1972.

Cracknell DG, ed. *Obligations: The law of tort*, 3rd ed. London: Old Bailey Press, 2004.

Crown Proceedings Act (CPA) 1947.

Davies M 2nd ed Textbook on Medical Law, Oxford University Press, Oxford, 1998.

De Than C and Shorts E. *Human rights*, 3rd ed. Harlow: Pearson Education Limited, 2013.

Donoghue v Stevenson HL [1932] HL All ER Repl.

Elliot C and Quinn F. *Tort law*, 7th ed. Harlow: Person Longman, 2009.

European Convention on Human Rights 1950.

European Withdrawal Act 2018 (C16).

EU Data Protection Directive 1995.

Free Dictionary. Available online at: https://www.thefreedictionary.com/ (accessed 30th August 2019).

General Data Protection Regulation (GDPR) 2018.

GMC Good Medical Practice, General Medical Council, 2018. Available online at: https://www.gmc-uk.org/ (accessed on 20th June 2019).

Greater Glasgow Health Board v Doogan & Anor [2014] UKSC 68.

Hammurabi's Code. Available online at: https://hekint.org/2017/01/30/oaths-codes-and-charters-in-medicine-over-the-ages/ (accessed on 14th November 2019).

Harris J. *The value of life: An introduction to medical ethics*. London: Routledge and Kegan Paul, 1985.

Hinchcliff S, Norman S and Schrober J. *Nursing practice and healthcare*, 5th ed. London: Arnold, 2008.

Historic UK. Available online at: https://www.historic-uk.com/HistoryUK/HistoryofScotland/The-Auld-Alliance-France-Scotland/ (accessed on 3rd August 2019).

Hodgson J and Lewthwaite J. *Tort law*, 2nd ed. Oxford: Oxford University Press, 2007.

Human Fertilisation and Embryology Act 1991.

Human Rights Act 1998.

International council for nurses. Available online at: https://www.icn.ch/nursing-policy/nursing-definitions (accessed on 1st July 2013).

International Declaration on Human Rights 1948.

Johnson v Fourie [2011] EWHC 1062 (QB).

Kituma v Nursing and Midwifery Council (Rev 1) [2009] EWHC 373.

Limitation Act 1980.

Makkan S. *The Human Rights Act 1998*. London: Callow Publishing, 2000.

Mason JK, McCall RA and Laurie GT. *Law and medical ethics*, 8th ed. London: Butterworths, 2010.

McDermitt T, ed. *Summa Theologiae: A concise translation*. Christian Classics, 1997.

McHale J and Tingle J. 3rd ed. *Law and nursing*. Oxford: Butterworth Heinemann, 2007.

Ministry of Justice. *Making sense of human rights: A short introduction*. Available online at: www.justice.gov.uk/aboutdocs/act-studyguide.pdf, 2006.

Montgomery v Lanarkshire Health Board [2015] UKSC 11.

NHS Claims. Available online at: https://nhsclaim.org.uk/?gclid=Cj0KCQjw2K3rBRDi-ARIsAOFSW_7wLAnbj5yxAQ57pRy2DhVd4tVMNbF3pErAGuU_-S8-e_Lql8eutssaAm-bEALw_wcB (accessed 30th August 2019).

NHS Constitution, © Crown copyright 2019, CCS0218952898 January 2019, Department of Health and Social Care, 2019.

NHS Trust A v M and NHS Trust B v H [2001] Fam 348.

Nicolson JB and Erskine J. An institute of the law of Scotland by John Erskine 1695–1768. Call Number: D 348 ERS, 1871.

NMC Code (2018) Professional standards of practice and behaviour for nurses, midwives and nursing associates. Available online at: https://www.nmc.org.uk/standards/code/ (accessed on 30th August 2019).

Nursing and Midwifery Order, 2001.

Prescription and Limitation Act 1973.

RCN. *Human rights and nursing: RCN position statement.* London: Royal College of nursing (RCN), 2012.

R v Allitt, 1992 [2007] EWHC 2845 (QB).

R v Instan [1893] 1 QB at 45.

Sidaway v. Bethlem Royal Hospital and Ors. [1985] AC 871; [1985] 1 All ER 643.

Singer P, in Silberbauer G, eds. *A companion to ethics.* Oxford: Blackwell Publishing, 2003.

Thompson M. *Ethics,* London: Hodder and Stoughton, 2003.

Wacks R. *Understanding jurisprudence: An introduction to legal theory,* 5th ed. Oxford: Oxford University Press, 2017.

Wilsher v Essex Area Health Authority [1987] QB 730.CA, 1988 AC 1074.

From beginning of life to adulthood

Chapter outline

Introduction
Human life and legal terminations
Child's welfare and best interests
Parental responsibility and minors
Age of criminal responsibility
Consent
Child abuse and safeguarding
Conclusion

Introduction

This chapter will consider the development of human rights, starting from the beginning of life to adulthood. The implications of abortions and the rights of the foetus are also considered.

The reality of a caring relationship is one based on trust and inevitably inequality. This is even more unbalanced for a developing human being who is vulnerable from the earliest stages of life. The concept of 'beginnings of life' alludes to the process and attempts to define the point at which life begins. Within various relevant disciplines, there is no consensus on when life begins. Sperm and a zygote can both be defined as living organisms. Does human life, then, begin with fertilization and the existence of an embryo? A question may also arise on defining the end of human life at the other end of the spectrum. Where death is concerned, the meaning of life may be more definitive unless a person is progressively in a persistent vegetative state or there is death of the brain or organ failure. The question arises: at what stage should an unborn being acquire human rights, and should this be on conception or birth? The role of the law is to define fundamental human rights. Moral values of a given society are also a focal point of the debate on the right to life. Ethics as well as religious values and science raise questions on the rights of the foetus vis-à-vis those of the mother (Brazier and Cave, 2016). Answers are not always obvious in ethical debates. The law, however, defines this as

3) In subsection (2), for paragraph (a) substitute—
"(a) references to embryos the creation of which was brought about in vitro (in their application to those where fertilisation or any other process by which an

embryo is created is complete) are to those where fertilisation or any other process by which the embryo was created began outside the human body whether or not it was completed there, and".

(Section 4, Human Fertilisation and Embryology Act 2008)

A different set of complex legal rules which are found in a number of statutes is applicable for life in the early stages and minors. Prior to current key UK legislation, the set of applicable rules was less clear when dealing with children. The term 'paramountcy of the welfare of the child' or sometimes called 'welfare principle' was first defined under the Children Act 1989. The focus of the discussion will be on treatment decisions, capacity and consent as well as safeguarding issues.

Human life and legal terminations

Article 2: Right to life, Human Rights Act 1998 is applicable to abortion
1. Everyone's right to life shall be protected by law. No one shall be deprived of his life intentionally save in the execution of a sentence of a court following his conviction of a crime for which the penalty is provided by law.

The above human right was tested in the *Paton v. United Kingdom, App. No. 8416/78, 3 Eur. H.R. Rep. 408 (1980),* where a husband contended that the foetus his wife was carrying at the time had the right to life and argued that termination of the pregnancy under the Abortion Act 1967 would go against and in breach of Article 2 of the Human Rights Act 1998. Mr Paton also argued that his own rights had been breached under Article 8, right to privacy. The European Commission on Human Rights found that the life of the foetus is intimately connected with, and cannot be regarded in isolation of, the life of the pregnant woman.

Box 3.1 Case: Paton v. United Kingdom European Commission of Human Rights 13 May 1980 (1981) 3 E.H.R.R. 408 Application No. 8416/78

The applicant, a UK citizen, was a married man who applied for an injunction to stop his wife from having an abortion at eight weeks.
    The 'life' of the foetus is intimately connected with, and cannot be regarded in isolation from, the life of the pregnant woman.

Box 3.2 Thinking point

Ms A, a 50-year-old single parent, has been informed by C, her 16-year-old daughter who recently received a firm offer for a place at a top university and is due to attend that university to study for a degree in law in two months' time, that she is eight weeks pregnant. Ms A, who has been saving up and is prepared to finance her daughter, becomes distraught, and the two have a showdown. Ms A threatens to cut her daughter off financially and throws her out, and she becomes homeless. The daughter is admitted to A&E after taking a paracetamol overdose and says she does not want the baby as she is not sure who the father is, and this will ruin her career. She is treated for anxiety and says she now wants an abortion so she can get on with her studies.

1   Consider C's rights under the Abortion Act 1967 in order to be allowed a legal abortion.
2   Can A, the mother, over-ride her daughter as she now says that, due to religious grounds, she (the mother) will look after the baby?

The enactment of the Universal Declaration of Human Rights (UDHR) 1945 resulted in its adoption by the United Nations General Assembly (A/RES/217, 10 December 1948 at Palais de Chaillot, following the Second World War. In respect of children the United Nations attempted to further fill a gap in legislation and develop an international treaty to protect the rights of the child, The Convention on the Rights of the Child, General Assembly resolution 44/25 of 20 November 1989, from 2 September 1990, Article 49:

Article 1 (definition of the child) Everyone under the age of 18 has all the rights in the Convention.

Article 2 (non-discrimination) The Convention applies to every child without discrimination, whatever their ethnicity, gender, religion, language, abilities or any other status, whatever they think or say, whatever their family background.

Article 3 (best interests of the child) The best interests of the child must be a top priority in all decisions and actions that affect children.

Article 4 (implementation of the Convention) Governments must do all they can to make sure every child can enjoy their rights by creating systems and passing laws that promote and protect children's rights.

Article 6 (life, survival and development) Every child has the right to life. Governments must do all they can to ensure that children survive and develop to their full potential.

(https://www.unicef.org.uk/what-we-do/un-convention-child-rights/)

The point at which life begins has been the focus of the development of child-related legislation for some time. Unfortunately, there is no complete agreement between disciplines such as medicine (and allied healthcare professions), philosophy, science, religion or ethics. The role of the law was to define this. Under the law the rights of the child are realized on birth. Under current legislation, the Abortion Act 1967 provides for, a mother may choose to have an abortion. This is subject to the Infant Life (Preservation) Act 1929 of England and Wales, to "destroy the life of a child capable of being born alive" if this is intentional termination outside the provisions of the Abortion Act. The maximum time set for legal termination is set at 23 weeks and 6 days of pregnancy, subject to the Abortion Act 1967. The grounds for abortion in UK law are provided for in Sections 58 and 59, of the Abortion Action Act 1967. Up to 24 weeks if there is any risk of harm to the mother of any of her existing children. The rationale was that abortions would be permissible as a child was not capable of being born.

- to prevent grave harm to the mental/physical health of the mother;
- to reduce the risk to the mother's life;
- if the baby will be 'seriously handicapped'.

(Section 59, Abortion Act 1967)

In 2014, 184,571 abortions were performed in England and Wales (DH, Abortion Statistics, England and Wales, 2014 [2015]). Department of Health and Social Care (2017) statistics also show that a total of 192,900 abortions were carried out for women who were resident in England and Wales in 2017 and as many as 197,533 abortions also including non-residents. The number and rate of terminations of pregnancy in Scotland in 2018 were at a ten-year high: There were 13,286 terminations (A National Statistics Publication for Scotland [2018]). Illegal abortions are outlawed in criminal law under Section 13 of the Offences against the Person Act 1861. There are two areas of the law where healthcare professionals may legally raise conscientious objection to participation, on the grounds of religion or other personal grounds.

As a legal principle, the UK is informed by the landmark US Supreme Court case, *Roe v Wade [1973] 410 US 113*, which, though not binding in the UK, is persuasive. Judge Blackmun ruled that 'We need not resolve the difficult question of when life begins. When those trained in the respective disciplines of medicine, philosophy, and theology are unable to arrive at any consensus, the judiciary, at this point in the development of man's knowledge, is not in a position to speculate as to the answer' (*R v Wade (1973) paragraph X*). This upheld a woman's right to have a termination and explored fundamental ethical issues and human rights related to abortion. It overturned previous decisions establishing a woman's right to choose to have an abortion. Previously abortions were permissible only to save a woman's life. The facts of *Roe v. Wade, 410 U.S. 113 (1973)* follow below:

> the Supreme Court held that a pregnant woman has a constitutional right, under the Fourteenth Amendment, to choose to terminate her pregnancy before viability as part of her freedom of personal choice in family matters.
> (http://www.bbc.co.uk/ethics/abortion/legal/roewade.shtml)

The question which arises is at what point the life of a foetus begins and whether it attains any rights. Based on current UK legislation, the Abortion Act 1973 allows for termination up to 24 weeks (please see above). Until recently, Northern Ireland was an exception, though women were open to travelling to other parts of the UK for terminations. Failure to comply with the law may have resulted in a criminal prosecution subject to Section 59 of the Offences Against the Person Act (OAPA) 1861.

Box 3.3 Case: R v Ahmed (Ajaz) [2010] EWCA Crim 1949

A man was charged with 'procuring a miscarriage' after taking his non-English speaking wife to a clinic for an abortion, having deceived her as to the nature of the procedure. A health professional subsequently communicate with the woman and ascertained that she did not consent.

http://www.parliament.scot/S5_JusticeCommittee/Inquiries/DA-Neal.pdf

A person may be charged under Section 58 OAPA 1861 if they procure an illegal abortion. Charges which may arise are abortion or child destruction. 'Any person who, with intent to destroy the life of a child capable of being born alive, by any wilful act causes a child to die before it has an existence independent of its mother, shall be guilty of an offence' (s1(1) Infant Life (Preservation) Act 1929).

If the child in question is under the age of 12 months, this means that the woman is guilty of infanticide.

Section1, Infanticide Act 1938, Offence of infanticide.
(1) Where a woman by any wilful act or omission causes the death of her child being a child under the age of twelve months, but at the time of the act or omission the balance of her mind was disturbed by reason of her not having fully recovered from the effect of giving birth to the child or by reason of the effect of lactation consequent upon the birth of the child, then, [if] the circumstances were such that but for this Act the offence would have amounted to murder [or manslaughter].
(https://www.legislation.gov.uk/ukpga/Geo6/1-2/36/section/1)

Nevertheless, prior to the Abortion Act (AA) 1967, there were also exceptions of legally justifiable abortions, one of which was in cases of rape. One such example was the Bourne Case, a leading case discussed below.

Before the AA 1967 Act: In cases of rape:

Box 3.4 Case: R v Bourne [1938] 3 All ER 615

A 14-year-old girl was a victim of multiple rapes (by several soldiers), and she subsequently fell pregnant. A gynaecologist performed an abortion on her and was charged with the offence of conducting an illegal abortion. He was acquitted. Mr Justice Macnaghten ruled that

> If the doctor is of the opinion, on reasonable grounds and with adequate knowledge, that the probable consequence of the continuance of the pregnancy will be to make the woman a physical or mental wreck, the jury are entitled to take the view that the doctor is operating for the purpose of preserving the life of the mother.

UK Key legislation related to Conception and Abortion are mainly regulated by two statutes, Human Embryology and Fertilisation Act 1990 and Abortion Act, 1967. These statutes also provide for conscientious objection. The legal conditions set by the Abortion Act are set out as follows:

(a) that the pregnancy has not exceeded its twenty-fourth week and that the continuance of the pregnancy would involve risk, greater than if the pregnancy were terminated, of injury to the physical or mental health of the pregnant woman or any existing children of her family; or
(b) that the termination is necessary to prevent grave permanent injury to the physical or mental health of the pregnant woman; or
(c) that the continuance of the pregnancy would involve risk to the life of the pregnant woman, greater than if the pregnancy were terminated; or

(d) that there is a substantial risk that if the child were born it would suffer from such physical or mental abnormalities as to be seriously handicapped.

(Section 1, Abortion Act 1967)

Illegal abortions are covered in criminal law under Section 13, Offences against the Person Act (OAPA) 1861. There are two areas of the law where healthcare professionals may legally raise a conscientious objection to participation in procedures, on the grounds of religion or other personal grounds. What happens when a healthcare professional objects to abortion on grounds of religion or other personal convictions?

Box 3.5 Royal College of Nursing v DHSS [1981] 2 WLR 279

Case law: conscientious objections

The Royal College of Nursing brought an action challenging the legality of the involvement of nurses in carrying out abortions. The Offences Against the Person Act 1861 makes it an offence for any person to carry out an abortion. The Abortion Act 1967 provided that it would be an absolute defence for a medically registered practitioner (i.e. a doctor) to carry out abortions, provided certain conditions were satisfied. Advances in medical science meant that surgical abortions were largely replaced with hormonal abortions, and it was common for these to be administered by nurses.

Held: It was legal for nurses to carry out such abortions. The act was aimed at doing away with backstreet abortions where no medical care was available. The actions of the nurses were therefore outside the mischief of the Offences Against the Person Act of 1861 and within the contemplate defence in the 1967 Act.

http://www.e-lawresources.co.uk/Royal-College-of-Nursing-v-DHSS.php

---

An individual woman who procures an illegal abortion may be may also be charged under Section 58, OAPA 1861 (above). The courts considered the rights of a married father in determining the right to abortion in the case below:

UK Key legislation related to Conception and Abortion are mainly regulated by two statutes, Human Embryology and Fertilisation Act 1990 and Abortion Act, 1967 (except where there is a threat to the mother's life). This has now changed in Northern Ireland under Section 9 of the Northern Ireland (Executive Formation etc) Act 2019 – with a new framework for access to abortion services in Northern Ireland. This is in line with the recommendations of the United Nations Committee 2018, on the Elimination of Discrimination Against Women Report.

The legal conditions set by the Abortion Act are set out as follows:

(a) that the pregnancy has not exceeded its twenty-fourth week and that the continuance of the pregnancy would involve risk, greater than if the pregnancy were terminated, of injury to the physical or mental health of the pregnant woman or any existing children of her family; or

(b) that the termination is necessary to prevent grave permanent injury to the physical or mental health of the pregnant woman; or

(c) that the continuance of the pregnancy would involve risk to the life of the pregnant woman, greater than if the pregnancy were terminated; or
(d) that there is a substantial risk that if the child were born it would suffer from
such physical or mental abnormalities as to be seriously handicapped.

(Section 1, Abortion Act 1967)

From an ethical perspective, healthcare professionals may 'wrestle with their conscience' as to whether they should participate in abortions or in human fertilization
procedures if they have strong views to the contrary, which may be based on religion
or other moral grounds. Are the courts sympathetic when a clinician has conscientious objections to participating in such procedures? A healthcare professional has
the onus to prove that they have conscientious grounds for objecting. In Scotland,
however, they need to demonstrate to the court, the role they play in abortions. The
law was insufficient to protect conscientious objections for two objectors who had
no direct involvement with abortions. The principle of the law is found in the following case;

**Box 3.6 Doogan & Anor v NHS Greater Glasgow & Clyde Health
Board [2013] ScotCS CSIH 36 (24 April 2013)**

Case: conscientious objection

Ms Doogan and Mrs Wood were employed as midwives in the labour ward at the respondents' Southern General Hospital and were also labour ward co-ordinators. Both
were practising Roman Catholics who, when they started working in the labour ward,
claimed conscientious objection to participation in terminations of pregnancy pursuant
to Section 4 of the Abortion Act 1967. The Supreme Court held that the right to conscientious objection did not extend to them as labour ward co-ordinators.

Under provisions of the AA 1967, the court interpreted the fact that the right to conscientious objection did not extend to those supervising other staff who were directly
involved in abortions. However, compare this with the following English case.

Child's welfare and best interests

A child's welfare must be paramount in any court decisions and 'the welfare checklist'
when dealing with a Children Act 1989 case. The court must pay regard to the following factors when making decisions for a child's welfare:

(a) The ascertainable wishes and feelings of the child concerned (considered in light
of their age and understanding);
(b) The child's physical, emotional and educational needs;
(c) The likely effect on the child of the change in circumstances;
(d) The child's age, sex, background and any characteristics which the court considers relevant;
(e) Any harm which the child has suffered or is at risk of suffering;

(f) How capable end of his parents, and any other person in relation to whom the court considers the question to be relevant is of meeting his needs;
(g) The range of owners open to the court under the Children Act 1989.

(Children Act 1989, s 1(3))

The paramountcy/welfare principle means that of the child should be the basis for court decisions in Family Law, under Section 1(3)(a) Children Act 1989. An example where this was established is the *Re P (Contact: Supervision) ([1996] 2 FLR 314 at p328*. This case concerned contact with absent parents. The court decision was that the interests of parents were secondary to those of a child. Furthermore, in *Re L (Contact: Genuine Fear) [2002] 1 FLR*, it was held that parents must have a burden of proof of the need for contact.

The Children Act 1989 focussed on the welfare of the child, and the Children Act 2004 enhanced the child's welfare and the principle of paramountcy of their welfare:

- a child's welfare is paramount when making any decisions about a child's upbringing, known as the "paramountcy principle"
- the court must ascertain the wishes and feelings of the child and shall not make an Order unless this is "better for the child than making no Order at all"
- every effort should be made to preserve the child's home and family links

(Section 1 "Paramountcy Principle", Children Act 2004)

Local authorities must not only support victims but also implement preventive measures for 'vulnerable' children with needs. The Sexual Offences Act 2003 applies.

Parental responsibility and minors

Article 3, UN Convention on the Rights of the Child (UNCRC), provides for the best interests of the child. Art 12 defines the rights of a 'mature' child who has the competence to have a degree of understanding in order to make informed decisions. They have a right to have their decision respected, UNICEF (1992).

The age of majority was reduced from 21 to 18, under the Children Act 2004 and the Childcare Act of 2006 applied reinforcing the focus on safeguarding and keeping the child safe. When a person reaches the age of 18, he attains majority, Family Law Reform Act 1969, c. 46, Section 1(1), he is deemed to be an adult in law. In England and Wales, the minimum age for marriage is 18. There are differences between Scotland and Northern Ireland, where the marriageable age is 16, with parental consent. Local authorities are required to keep in touch with vulnerable groups until at least the age of 21 (Children (Leaving Care) Act 2000).

The issues related to responsibility and the paramountcy/welfare (principle) of the child should be the basis for court decisions in family law:

– a child's welfare is paramount when making any decisions about a child's upbringing, known as the "paramountcy principle"
– the court must ascertain the wishes and feelings of the child and shall not make an Order unless this is "better for the child than making no Order at all"
– every effort should be made to preserve the child's home and family links

(Section 1(3) (a) Children Act 1989)

An example where this principle was applied is the *Re P (Contact: Supervision) ([1996] 2 FLR 314 at p328*. Regarding contact with absent parents, it was ruled that the interests of such a parent were secondary to the welfare of the child. In contrast, *Re L (Contact: Genuine Fear) [2002] 1 FLR* held that the burden is on the parent to prove the need for contact. The Family Law Reform Act 1969 defined the age of majority and presumed capacity of a child or adolescence. The law presumes that children below the age of majority have not attained the age of consent in most instances of consent. There are, however, exceptions when it comes to treatment, *Gillick v West Norfolk and Wisbech AHA [1986] AC 11*, on informed consent below.

Age of criminal responsibility

Responsibility, relates to accountability, and alludes to conduct mounting to a crime. A child aged 10 cannot be convicted of a criminal offence but may be placed under supervision *(Crime and Disorder Act 1998)*. At the age of 12, however, they may be placed under a detention and training order (for up to 24 months) for offences that would have incurred imprisonment if an adult *(Powers of Criminal Courts (Sentencing) Act 2000)*.

There was a presumption in law, under the long-standing principle of *doli incapax*, which meant that a child aged below 24 years lacks the criminal responsibility to commit a crime. This has, however, since changed due to a Government's response, in a White Paper entitled *Crime, Justice and Protecting the Public (1990, Cmnd 965) at para 8.4*, which proposed that "between the ages of 10 and 13 a child may only be convicted of a criminal offence if the prosecution can show that he knew that what he did was seriously wrong." This was applied in the James Bulger Case, in which a ten-year-old was convicted. At 17, people can be committed to a remand centre or prison. From the age of 18, they are likely to face criminal charges dealt with in adult courts.

Consent

In England and Wales, a child may be married at age 16, with parental consent (Marriage Act 1949 and Marriage (Same Sex Couples) Act 2013). A civil partnership was registerable at 16 (Civil Partnership Act 2004), and there has been a change since extending this to different sex partners, under the Civil Partnerships, Marriages and Deaths (Registration etc) Act 2019. Parental consent is no longer required for marriage, when both parties are 18 (Family Law Reform Act 1969). In Scotland, a child between the age of 16 and 18 can be married without the need for parental consent. Those from other parts of the UK may travel to Scotland to be married, without the need for parental consent and without a residence requirement. At the age 16, all sexual activities are permitted in law, provided that this is mutually consensual.

Regarding treatment decisions (the Family Law Reform Act 1969), a child who is aged 16 or older may give consent to treatment. Regarding medical treatment, there is a presumption that a child under the age of 16 is incompetent and that a person with parental responsibility has a duty to act in the child's best interests (Family Law Reform Act 1969). A young person over the age of 16 years can give a valid consent to surgical or medical treatment (Section 8(3) of the Family Law Reform Act 1969). If a child refuses treatment, a parent or court can over-ride the refusal.

Nevertheless, the bar has been 'lowered' as a child of a younger age may now be deemed to be competent, provided they have an adequate degree of understanding of the nature of treatment, the benefits and the risks (*Gillick v West Norfolk and Wisbech AHA [1986] AC 112*); please also see the case below.

Box 3.7 Case: Gillick V West Norfolk and Wisbech AHA [1986] AC 112 [1986] 1 FLR 224

A DHSS circular stated that in certain circumstances a doctor could lawfully prescribe contraception for a girl under 16 without the consent of the parents.

Mrs Gillick challenged this in the courts on religious grounds, arguing that children below the age of 16 were not competent to consent on their own behalf and that the circular adversely affected her ability to discharge her duties as a parent.

Held: A child who is deemed to be competent may make informed decisions on contraceptives. Lord Fraser stated that a doctor could proceed to give contraceptive advice and treatment to a girl under 16 (Lord Fraser Guidelines):

provided he is satisfied on the following matters:

1   that the girl (although under the age of 16 years of age) will understand his advice
2   that he cannot persuade her to inform her parents or to allow him to inform the parents that she is seeking contraceptive advice
3   that she is very likely to continue having sexual intercourse with or without contraceptive treatment
4   that unless she receives contraceptive advice or treatment her physical or mental health or both are likely to suffer
5   that her best interests require him to give her contraceptive advice, treatment or both without the parental consent

The case also established the Gillick Competence, which is tested based on their (child's) capacity to understand. Validity of consent depends on the mental capacity of child or parent giving the consent. For informed consent to be valid, the patient (applicable to child) must,

- be competent to take the particular decision;
- have received sufficient information to take it; and
- not be acting under duress.

(DoH, 2003)

Furthermore, Article 12 of the United Nations Convention on the Rights of the Child 1989, the views of the child, requires that 'Every child has the right to express their views, feelings and wishes in all matters affecting them, and to have their views considered and taken seriously'.

It is important that the information provided should be in a format that the child can understand, and that the child's understanding is checked by the person who is obtaining the consent.

Child abuse and safeguarding

Safeguarding is a matter of concern regarding safety of vulnerable children who may be at risk. There is some leeway in that not only children but also young adults or adolescents up to the age of 19 are protected by the law. In the case of those with learning disabilities, the upper age limit of 24 is set. The court may appoint a supervisor to keep an eye on vulnerable children, under Section 35, 36, Children Act 1989. The Social Care Act 2014 places a legal duty on Local authorities to minimize risk for vulnerable people in the community with disabilities and long-term conditions.

The classification or types of child abuse, though similar to adult abuse in many ways, are identified below and may include physical, psychological and sexual exploitation (via direct or online grooming); also included is the concept of modern-day slavery, which is achieved through human trafficking. This is now recognized in the Department of Education safeguarding guidelines below. Child abuse may take many forms and is much broader than previously thought, with a broader definition of abuse:

> 12. Children may be vulnerable to neglect and abuse or exploitation from within their family and from individuals they come across in their day-to-day lives. These threats can take a variety of different forms, including sexual, physical and emotional abuse; neglect; exploitation by criminal gangs and organised crime groups; trafficking; online abuse; sexual exploitation and the influences of extremism leading to radicalisation.
>
> (Working Together to Safeguard Children, 2018)

Safeguarding should be achieved through risk assessment, and risk management by putting in place, preventive measures and support. This may include vulnerable children with needs being placed under a care order or supervision. The Social Care Act 2017 was aimed at improving the welfare of children in care and aligning safeguarding, with the updated 'Working together to safeguarding Children (2018)'. One new key provision to the Children Act 1989; one aspect is the extension of entitlement to a Personal Advisor (PA) beyond the age of 21 to all care leavers up to 25 years old. A Local authority shares parental responsibility with the parents. It can place restrictions on parental responsibility, and can remove the child from care, but the parents can still usually consent to treatment. Where a vulnerable child is at risk, the Local council Social services may apply for a care order, a court can create a care order under Section 31(1) (a) of the Children Act, '… placing a child in the care of a designated local authority, with parental responsibility being shared between the parents and the local authority'.

Box 3.8 Thinking point

B, an eight-year-old girl, attends A&E with a fractured wrist, which the mother says she sustained after an accidental fall at home. She also has what appears to be a large bruise on her forehead. They are also accompanied by a 30-year-old man, who tells the receptionist that he is the father. The man smells of alcohol. He is loud, argumentative and keeps threatening the mother. The woman seems to be submissive and uncomfortable with the male.

The nurse asks to speak to the child on her own, and B admits that she is terrified of the man, who is actually her mum's boyfriend, and says that earlier that day he had slapped her across the face and pushed her so she fell over. This occurred after she had not made her bed. She admits that such violent behaviour happens often.

1   What action (s) should the nurse take?
2   What does the NMC Code (2018) require on safeguarding vulnerable children?

The Children Act 2004 also includes support for the broader category of children staying safe. Child Care Act 2006 imposes a statutory duty of care on Local authorities and this requires them to safeguard vulnerable children. The Royal College of Nursing guidelines for safeguarding vulnerable people including children require the nurse to;

- *Identify* safeguarding concerns.
- *Report* the concerns – for most nurses, midwives, health visitors and HCAs this will be in conjunction with partner agencies and you should use organisational and local policies.
- *Participate* in enquiries, debriefing and (where appropriate) in developing a protection plan.
- *Reflect* on the outcomes and learning.

(RCN, https://www.rcn.org.uk/clinical-topics/safeguarding)

Box 3.9 Thinking point: a key case law review

There are several cases of child abuse, and what they have in common is health and safety issues. It is often the case that systemic weaknesses are present, and practices are unsafe, resulting in harm to children.

1   Victoria Climbié

She was born in the Ivory Coast and then moved to France to live with her aunt, ostensibly to receive a good education. The French authorities had concerns about the child's absenteeism from school but never got a chance to act on this as the auntie moved to London. The abuse started as verbal and emotional but soon escalated to physical after the auntie moved in with her lover. Victoria was forced to sleep in a bath with her hands tied up with masking tape and forced to eat like a dog. She was beaten up. She was admitted with injuries and malnutrition and diagnosed with multiple organ failure and 128 injuries.

The auntie and her lover were both convicted of murder and are serving a life sentence.

The Climbie Report, Health Foundation, https://navigator.health.org.uk, 2007.

Furthermore, The Climbie Inquiry held that

… was critical of the senior managers and senior members of authorities who had responsibility for the strategic oversight of services for children. Lord Laming suggested that a number of the agencies were underfunded, inadequately staffed and poorly led. The inquiry made general criticisms of basic procedures such as comprehensive record-keeping and information sharing and suggested that there had been 'widespread organisational malaise'.

(The Climbie Report, Health Foundation, 2007)

The Children Act 2004 subsequently implemented the main changes which included getting rid of child protection registers which were replaced by child protection plans and creating an integrated children's computer system (ICS). The aim was to ensure improved sharing of information between interested parties. Other high-profile cases which have highlighted similar concern and a system failure on the part of individuals and organizations and therefore letting down the vulnerable child, the *Re: Baby P* (Community Care, 2017).

Nowadays, vulnerable children who have access to the internet are also more likely to be at risk of being groomed, through surfing on the internet and through social media. Peer pressure may contribute to a culture which sees vulnerable children falling foul of paedophiles directly or via online. The NSPCC indicates the following statistics.

- 16 per cent of surveyed primary school-aged children and 19 per cent of surveyed secondary school students said they had seen content which encouraged people to hurt themselves.
- 11- to 18-year-olds reported seeing sexual content in 16 per cent of reviews of the most popular social networks, apps and games.
- 31 per cent of children aged 12 to 15 reported seeing worrying or nasty online content.

(NSPCC, How safe are our children? 2019)

Conclusion

Health and social care staff have a duty of care in ethics and in law to always act in the child's best interest, the welfare principle must be applied by the courts in family law cases. The question of beginnings and right to life in this area can be contentious and may be contentious for a long time, whether life should be preserved at all costs or if there are exceptions. The rights of the unborn child may be seen as competing against those of the mother in cases where the life of the mother may be at risk, or where the quality of life is deemed to be unacceptable quality with serious physical or genetic risks, or the result of a crime (rape, incest). Ethical issues arise and questions may be asked.

Children are even more vulnerable than adults, and in cases of abuse, there is a need to safeguard and protect those rights, especially in the area of the human rights of the child. Abuse may take place at the hands of those who children should trust. Health and social care staff should recognize signs of abuse, and where there are concerns, concerns about vulnerable children should be raised with the social care departments of Local authorities. It is better for them to occasionally get it wrong than to do nothing with the result of a child falling victim to abuse. The reasons for abuse of children may be varied, though they can often be related: for example, mental health or substance misuse issues and parents or guardians with a history of violence can be risk factors. Social deprivation and poverty are another possibility which have been linked to abuse (Lefebre et al., 2017), though child abuse is not necessarily limited to poor households. Child abuse may or may not reflect the family background or history of the perpetrators.

Legislation is critical in defining and applying human rights form the beginning of life and safeguarding the best interests of children. Procedures, however, are as good as the people who follow them and if implemented can be effective in protecting the rights of the child.

References

Abortion Act 1967.

Abortion Act 1967, Sections 58 and 59.

BBC Online, Ethics. Available online at: http://www.bbc.co.uk/ethics/abortion/legal/roewade. shtml (accessed on 13th May 2019).

Children Act 2004, Section 1.

Children (Leaving Care) Act 2000.

Civil Partnerships Marriages and Deaths Act 2019.

Civil Partnership Act 2004.

Climbie Report, Health Foundation (2007) Available online at: https://navigator.health.org.uk (accessed on 2nd December 2019).

Crime and Disorder Act 1998.

Crime, Justice and Protecting the Public (1990, Cmnd 965) at para 8.4.

Department of Education Guidance. Working together to safeguard children A guide to inter-agency working to safeguard and promote the welfare of children, July 2018. Available on-line at: https://assets.publishing.service.gov.uk/government/uploads/system/uploads/attach-ment_data/file/779401/Working_Together_to_Safeguard-Children.pdf (accessed on 21st November 2019).

Department of Health (2003) Good practice in consent: Implementation guide for health care professionals. Available online at: https://www.health-ni.gov.uk/sites/default/files/publica-tions/dhssps/good-practice-consent.pdf (accessed on 1st June 2019).

Department of Health and Social Care (2017) Abortion statistics, England and Wales, 2014. Available online at: https://www.gov.uk/government/statistics/report-on-abortion-statistics-in-england-and-wales-for-2014 (accessed on 19th March 2019).

Department of Health and Social Care (2017) Abortion statistics, England and Wales: 2017 sum-mary information from the abortion notification forms returned to the Chief Medical Officers of England and Wales. Available online at: www.gov.uk/dh (accessed on 30th March 2019).

Family Law Reform Act 1969, section 1(1), section 8(3).

Gillick v West Norfolk and Wisbech AHA [1986] AC 11.

Human Fertilisation and Embryology Act 1990.

Human Fertilisation and Embryology Act 2008, Section 4.

Human Rights Act 1998, Article 2.

Infant Life (Preservation) Act 1929.

Lefebre R, Fallon B, Van Wert M and Filippelli J. Examining the relationship between eco-nomic hardship and child maltreatment using data from the Ontario incidence study of re-ported child abuse and neglect-2013 (OIS-2013), 2017.

Life (Preservation) Act 1929.

Marriage Act 1949.

Marriage (Same Sex Couples) Act 2013.

National Statistics Publication for Scotland (2018) Available online at: https://www.isdscot land.org/Health-Topics/Sexual-Health/Publications/2019-05-28/2019-05-28-Termina-tions-2018-Report.pdf (accessed on 2nd June 2019).

NSPCC, how safe are our children? (2019) Online abuse an overview of data on child abuse online. Available online at: https://learning.nspcc.org.uk/media/1747/how-safe-are-our-children-2019.pdf (accessed on 20th July 2019).

Offences Against the person Act 1861, Section 13.

Paton v United Kingdom. App. No 8416/78.

Powers of Criminal Courts (Sentencing Act 2000).

R v Ahmed (Ajaz) [2010] EWCA Crim 1949.

R v Bourne [1938] 3 All ER 615.

Re L Contact: Genuine [2002]1FLR.

Re P (Contact Supervision) [1996] 2.

Re Baby P. Available online at: https://www.communitycare.co.uk/2017/08/03/ten-years-baby-p-social-works-story/ (accessed on 3rd August 2019).

Roe v. Wade, 410 U.S. 113, 1973.

Royal College of Nursing v DHSS [1981] 2 WLR 279.

Royal College of Nursing, Guidance on Safeguarding (2019) Available online at: https://www.rcn.org.uk/clinical-topics/safeguarding (accessed on 7th August 2019).

Section 4, Human Fertilisation and Embryology Act 2008. Available online at: https://www.legislation.gov.uk/ukpga/2008/22/section/1

Social Care Act 2014.

United Nations Convention on the Rights of the Child (UNCRC), Article 3, 1992.

United Nations Committee 2018, on the Elimination of Discrimination against Women Report.

Working together to safeguarding children (2018) A guide to inter-agency working to safeguard and promote the welfare of children Available online at: https://www.gov.uk/government/publications/working-together-to-safeguard-children--2 (accessed on 12th September 2019).

Confidentiality, information and technology

Chapter outline

Introduction
Confidentiality, the legal framework
Communication, record-keeping
Development of data protection, case law
Information technology and artificial intelligence (AI)
Conclusion
Reference

Introduction

There are various aspects of patient information. This includes verbal and written formats, which requires accurate record-keeping, which is important for effective treatment and continuity of care and is evidence of the care which was provided. All the data and medical information related to patient care is a key source. This all relates to communication which is at the heart of the care delivery. This is related to ongoing record of diagnosis and patient treatment information which is found in the patient's records. This also helps in maintaining continuity of care as an opportunity to evaluate the effectiveness of the interventions. The courts will not look sympathetically towards a defence in a clinical negligence case where there is a lack or poor record-keeping, as they will require evidence for proof of the care that was given. This may also be used as evidence in a case of litigation. If it is not documented, it doesn't exist. This was the view in *Miller & Another v Health Service Commissioner for England [2018] EWCA Civ 144*, the Court of Appeal considered a decision made by the Health Service Commissioner for England in relation to a complaint about medical treatment. Gloster LJ referred in her judgment to *'an unfortunate use of language'* on behalf of the Commissioner's Director:

> ... when he said "if it is not written down it didn't happen unless there is other corroborating evidence"

This is clearly linked to information technology, which is an important facet of patient information, involving record-keeping of results of investigations and ongoing treatment. The role of information technology and artificial intelligence should not be underestimated. In computer-aided diagnosis, 'The computer output is used as a "second opinion" in assisting radiologists' image interpretations. The computer algorithm generally consists of several steps that may include image processing, image feature analysis' (Shiraishi et al., 2011, p 449). This means that treatment can be delivered more effectively if this is utilized in the right way. A duty of confidentiality is implied under data protection legislation in order to ensure the safety of otherwise sensitive patient-identifiable information. Ethical considerations may also arise when the application of technology and artificial intelligence is considered.

Confidentiality, the legal frameworks

A nurse is privy to confidential and/or sensitive information related to a patient medical and social history, without the need to acquire a patient's consent. This is due to a fiduciary relationship, which is based on trust. This means that there is an imbalance of power, control and dependence on the part of a patient. Most patients are vulnerable due to their condition.

In common law, and in providers owe a duty of care to the

(1) any person making a request for information to a public authority is entitled –
(a) to be informed in writing by the public authority whether it holds information of the description specified in the request, and
(b) if that is the case, to have that information communicated to him.

(Freedom of Information Act 2003)

A health record includes confidential information which is related to a person's health, and this includes both physical and mental aspects. As part of the common law duty of care to the patient *Donoghue v Stevenson* [1932] AC 562 (HL), the nurse must ensure that any patient-identifiable information which comes into their hands in the course of their employment is secured and remains confidential. In a therapeutic relationship, legislation also requires a duty of confidentiality stating that 'patient information may not be shared with others except on a need to know basis without the patient's consent, except as provided for by, Schedules 2 and 3 of the Data Protection Act 1998 and General Data Protection Regulation, 2018.

It stands to reason that the nurse owes the service user a duty of confidence or confidentiality arising from this relationship of trust and that the nurse may not breach that confidence by passing on this confidential information to a third party with no. Patient information may only be divulged to other healthcare professionals on a need to know basis. unless this is on a need-to-know basis only. It stands to reason that a healthcare professional owes the service users a duty of care (confer in Chapter 2) to ensure that patients are not harmed by nurses' negligent actions of commission or omission. This duty of care arises when a patient discloses information to a clinician, based on trust – in such circumstances it is reasonable to that the information will be held in confidence.

a) is a legal obligation that is derived from case law;
b) is a requirement established with professional codes of conduct; and
c) must be included within NHS employment contracts as a specific requirement linked to disciplinary procedures.

(Department of Health 2003)

What are health records? This includes wide range of information which is related to care and informing on their progress, vital signs, result of investigations and records of medications administered. A patient or their representative may have access to their Access to Health Records Act 1990 regulated access to health records and '... provides certain individuals with a right of access to the health records of a deceased individual';

> Section 3(1)(f) of that Act as, 'the patient's personal representative and any person who may have a claim arising out of the patient's death'. A personal representative is the executor or administrator of the deceased person's estate.
> (Access to Health Records Act (AHRA) 1990)

Access to information should be controlled and limited to those on a need to know basis. This is based on 'the power', control or influence that the nurse may have over vulnerable older patients. This power may be abused, breaching the human rights of a vulnerable older person. There is a legal requirement maintaining confidentiality, which is a basic Human Rights;

> 1 Everyone has the right to respect for his private and family life, his home and his correspondence.
> 2 There shall be no interference by a public authority with the exercise of this right except such as is in accordance with the law and is necessary in a democratic society in the interests of national security, public safety or the economic well-being of the country, for the prevention of disorder or crime, for the protection of health or morals, or for the protection of the rights and freedoms of others.
> (Article 8, Human Rights Act 1998)

Section 3 of the Public Records Act 1958 (Public Records (Scotland) Act 1937, Public Records Act (Northern Ireland) 1923 and Government of Wales Act 1998) allows exceptions to disclosure of records. The NMC suggests that records may be disclosed on the following grounds:

> • if this is in the interest of public health as provided by statute,
> • for the protection of persons (including the patient) 'at risk of significant harm'
> • when ordered to do so by a court of law.

> (NMC, 2015)

There are more justifications for disclosure. Further to Section 60 of the Health and Social Care Act 2001, the Secretary of State for Health may authorize use of patient and authorized health service bodies to disclose patient-identifiable information. Section 61 of the same statute established the Patient Information Advisory Group to monitor use of patient information. This includes data which is patient identifiable if this is deemed necessary for supporting essential national Health Service (NHS) activity or if this is in the public interest. More examples will be considered below.

There are exception to disclosures, as required by statute. Examples are the Road Traffic Act 1988 requirement for disclosure of confidential information, for example if a driver was intoxicated. Also, under the Terrorism Prevention and Investigation

Measures Act 2011, healthcare professionals are obliged to report or disclose any action of preparation or execution of terrorism. Another example is subject to the Criminal Appeal Act 1995, if a crime has been committed, is suspected or evidently about to be committed. In cases of Public Health Control of Disease) Act 1984, there is clearly a public interest which overrides the need for a duty of confidentiality on information related to an individual. NMC Code of Professional Conduct and Ethics (2018) makes it clear that a fiduciary relationship means that the nurse must maintain confidentiality.

Further examples mean that the public interest overrides an individual interest,

Public Health (Control of Disease) Act 1984 and Public Health (Infectious Diseases) Regulations 1988 – Medical and public health nurses are required to notify the relevant local authority officer, if they suspect a patient of having a notifiable disease.

Box 4.1 Thinking point

An 18-year-old male is admitted to A&E late one night with a severe laceration to his leg. He claims that he sustained this while jumping over a barbed wire fence with friends taking a shortcut.

One hour later, while he is being treated, two police officers enter the department, stating that they are investigating a hit-and-run case by a stolen car, committed earlier in the night. They have a general description of the suspect driver, given to them by two passers-by who chased him off after running, and they also have samples of blood and torn clothing found on a fence near the scene. They demand access to the medical notes of all those fitting the description who entered A&E in the last three hours.

What would you do?

Consider:

1   Subject to *Police and Criminal Evidence Act (PACE) 1984* – the police can apply for a court order for accessing medical records for the purpose of crime investigation.

2   *Road Traffic Act 1988* – All citizens are required by law to provide the police, on request, with information (name, address) to identify a driver alleged to have committed a traffic offence.

Box 4.2 Case: W v. Edgell [1990] 1 ALL ER 835

W was a prisoner in a secure hospital following convictions for killing five people and wounding several others. He made an application to a mental health tribunal to be transferred to a regional unit. An independent psychiatrist, Dr Edgell, was asked by W's legal advisors to provide a confidential expert opinion that they hoped would show that W was no longer a danger to the public. However, Dr Edgell was of the opinion that in fact W was still dangerous. W's application was withdrawn. Dr Edgell, knowing that his opinion would not be included in the patient's notes, sent a copy to the medical director of the hospital and to the Home Office.

The patient brought an action for breach of confidence.

The Court of Appeal held that the breach was justified in the public interest, on grounds of protection of the public from dangerous criminal acts. However, the Court said the risk must be 'real, immediate and serious'.

There are exceptions where the information is related to counter fraud, where disclosure of relevant aspects of patient information may be permissible, under the NHS Act 2006. Furthermore, in employment law, most employers will require a confidentiality clause in the contract of employment. This means that healthcare employees may not divulge confidential information without risking breaching their contract of employment. Litigation for defamation or libel (Scotland) is subject to the United Kingdom Defamation Acts 1996 and 2013. Healthcare providers have a duty of care in ethics and in law to respect this confidentiality. From an ethical perspective, this is a reasonable expectation within a fiduciary relationship. Under the Defamation Act 2013, a wronged client or service whose trust is betrayed by a professional who breaches confidentiality by disclosing person-identifiable information may be entitled to recover damages in a civil court. However, disclosure without the user's consent may be permissible in law, '... patient information may not be passed on to others without the patient's consent except as permitted under Schedule 2 and 3 of the Data Protection Act 1998, or where applicable, under the common law where there is an overriding public interest' (DoH [1996] the Protection and Use of Patient Information: Guidance from the Department of Health HSG (1996, p. 18).

Communication and record-keeping

Any team of professionals needs effective communication in order to function effectively. Communication involves the exchange of ideas or passing on information through conversation and sharing information as well as having a two-way dialogue (Adair, 1984). This dialogue exists between healthcare professionals and a patient as well as between colleagues and members of the multi-disciplinary team. It has been further suggested that communication involves both 'a monologue' and 'a dialogue' (Adair, 1984, p. 154). This may apply to reflection. Records are the outward evidence of communication and of the care that has been provided. The generation and maintenance of good quality records can be evidence of the provision of good quality care. Multi-disciplinary teams of professionals caring for the same group of patients will benefit from sharing good communication in the form of records, whether verbal or written. The latter nevertheless has the advantage of being more reliable, as it is permanent. Another underlying rationale for ensuring quality record-keeping is as evidence of,

- high standards of clinical care,
- continuity of care,
- better communication and dissemination of information between members of the
- interprofessional healthcare team, an accurate account of the treatment and care planning and delivery,
- the ability to detect (and monitor) problems, such as changes in the patient's or client's condition, at an early stage.

(NMC, 2015)

Due to the importance of the nature of their work, nurses and other healthcare professionals must justify this by accurate documentation of communication. Verbal or unwritten information is not reliable as mistakes can be made and people are more likely to forget and in time, the message may become distorted. Any set standards, found in both national and local guidance, must be followed. Many systems of work usually have their own relevant formats or templates (with certain criteria required), such as frameworks or tools for ease of information gathering: for example for carrying out nursing assessments documentation.

Recording of any professional care activities and related communication should therefore be informative and accurate for it to have any meaningful effect on care.

The RCN (2017) summarized the key principles of record-keeping as follows:

Key principles

- Records should be completed at the time or as soon as possible after the event.
- All records must be signed, timed and dated if handwritten. If digital, they must be traceable to the person who provided the care that is being documented.
- Ensure that you are up to date in the use of electronic systems in your place of work, including security, confidentiality and appropriate usage.
- Records must be completed accurately and without any falsification and provide information about the care given as well as arrangements for future and ongoing care.
- Jargon and speculation should be avoided.
- When possible, the person in your care should be involved in the record-keeping and should be able to understand what the records say.
- Records should be readable when photocopied or scanned.
- In the rare case of needing to alter a record, the original entry must remain visible (draw a single line through the record) and the new entry must be signed, timed and dated.
- Records must be stored securely and should only be destroyed following your local policy

(RCN, 2017)

The importance of effective communication in nursing is underpinned by the need for professionals who are responsible for care to share information with colleagues or other healthcare professionals providing direct or indirect care. This is vital for delivery of care, effectiveness and continuity.

Factor 1 Good practice should indicate that; communication is adapted to meet the needs of people, carers and groups. This includes consideration of their emotional state, hearing, vision and other physical and cognitive abilities and developmental needs, as well as their preferred language and possible need for an interpreter and translator

(DOH [2010] Essence of Care, in Buka et al. [2016, p. 102])

Record-keeping shows ongoing communication between the nurse and the patient and family, as well as healthcare professional colleagues. It is therefore important that this is done to a high standard. Any form of records may be subject to clinical audit and may be accessed by patients or their representatives as well by the employer in disciplinary cases. Most important of all, clinical records are necessary as a framework for nursing decision-making and for monitoring the patient's progress from an initial assessment and the care planning nursing process. Quality record-keeping should be at the heart of continuity of care and interaction between the patient and the nurse as well as the multi-disciplinary team. Nursing and other healthcare professionals need good record-keeping, demonstrating their 'professionalism' by maintaining a high standard of practice. Records may be called into evidence in a court of law. In a criminal prosecution, they may also be used by both sides in a civil litigation case. It is therefore important that patient records should

> Be factual, consistent and accurate.
> Be written as soon as possible after an event has occurred, providing current information on the care and condition of the patient.
> Be written clearly and in such a manner that the text cannot be erased.
> Be written in such a manner that any alterations or additions are dated, timed and signed in such a way that the original entry can be read clearly. and …
> Be accurately dated, timed and signed, with the signature printed alongside the first entry.
> Not include abbreviations, jargon, meaningless phrases, irrelevant speculation and offensive, subjective statements.
> Be readable on any photocopier.
>
> (NMC, 2009)

The Data Protection Act 1998/General has been updated by the Data Protection Regulation (GDPR) 2018 from May.

It is necessary for healthcare professionals who have access to patient-identifiable information to maintain this fiduciary trust-based relationship by ensuring confidentiality.

You should seek patients' and clients' wishes regarding sharing information with their family and others.

The main statutes regulating this area are the Data Protection Act (DPA) 1988, which regulated the storage of paper (both typed and handwritten) records, and the Data Protection Act (DPA) 1998 (which has largely replaced the 1988 Act), giving patients access to all personal data in general and electronic records specifically. Importantly, this statute also created the role of the Information Commissioner's Office (ICO), with one commissioner for England and Wales and one for Scotland and Northern Ireland each. The ICO has legal powers to enforce tighter controls and to ensure that organizations comply with the requirements of the DPA 1998. It is important to note that these powers are focussed on ensuring that organizations meet the obligations of the act. The data protection powers of the Information Commissioner's Office are to,

> • … conduct assessments to check organisations are complying with the Act;
> • serve information notices requiring organisations to provide the Information Commissioner's Office with specified information within a certain time period;
> • serve enforcement notices and 'stop now' orders where there has been a breach of the Act, requiring organisations to take (or refrain from taking) specified steps in order to ensure they comply with the law;
> • prosecute those who commit criminal offences under the (DPA) 1998 Act;

- conduct audits to assess whether organisations processing of personal data follows good practice; and
- to report to Parliament on data protection issues of concern.

(ICO, 2013)

The Access to Medical Records Act 1990 or Access to Health Records (Northern Ireland) Order 1993 which used to give a patient access to their records, has now been largely repealed and replaced by the DPA 1998, and covers only release of records in respect of deceased persons (where litigation may follow). Patient's representatives may be charged for access to records. Furthermore, under the DPA 1998, a patient or their representative has free access if they wish to view records only but is required to pay much for copies of manual records. The Freedom of Information (Scotland) Act 2002 applies. The Caldicott Report (1997) and its principles aimed at setting out the highest practical standards for handling confidential information, and therefore apply equally to all routine and ad hoc flows of patient information, whether clinical or non-clinical, in manual or electronic format. These must also be easily identifiable (HSC 1998/89), implementing the recommendations of the Caldicott Report (1997) which recommended further guidance in the area of record.

These principles, combined with national and local guidance, should provide a framework of quality standards. The security and safe storage of healthcare records should be the responsibility of locally appointed Caldicott guardians whose responsibility will be the management of confidentiality as well as access to personal information. These guidelines have since been adopted for safeguarding public records. The Freedom of Information Act 2000, giving access to information held by public authorities, may not be used for access to patient-identifiable information. The General Data Protection Regulations (2018) are found within The Data Protection Act 2018. This statute controls how personal information is used by organizations, including the NHS and other businesses.

Box 4.3 Thinking point

An 80-year-old man whose daughter lives in Australia is diagnosed with mild dementia, in the early stages of diagnosis and is admitted with pneumonia.
  Actions:

1   An informal carer and his wife, who are really neighbours, are the closest people who visit him and would like an update on his condition, though only the daughter's name is listed as next of kin.
2   What actions would you take, and how much information, if any, would you give him?

A duty of confidentiality is not absolute as there are exceptions. The general rule is to seek the patient's consent before disclosure:

Disclosure
27 Information that can identify a person in your care must not be used or disclosed for purposes other than healthcare without the individual's explicit consent. However, you can release this information if the law requires it, or where there is a wider public interest.

28 Under common law, you are allowed to disclose information if it will help to prevent, detect, investigate or punish serious crime or if it will prevent abuse or serious harm to others.

(NMC, 2015)

Good record-keeping means that the information is relevant comprehensive and the purpose of processing them legitimate. This is regulated by the Caldicott Principles are applicable to all types of records. The Caldicott Principles are summarized by the following principles.

Development of data protection, case law

The eight principles (of the Data Protection Act 1998) regulate the generation, processing and management of records:

1. Data must be processed fairly and lawfully.
2. Obtained for one or more specified and lawful purposes.
3. Personal data shall be adequate, relevant and not excessive.
4. Personal data shall be accurate and, where necessary, kept up to date.
5. Must not be kept for longer than is necessary.
6. Be compatible with the rights of data subjects.
7. Appropriate technological measures must be taken to safeguard the data.
8. Must not be transferred to a country or territory outside the European Economic Area, unless an adequate level of protection is in place.

(Data Protection Act 1998)

The general principle of confidentiality is based on the common law duty of care. Where there has been a breach; the owner of records can sue for defamation and damages where there has been unauthorized disclosure.

Box 4.4 Case: AG v Guardian Newspapers Ltd. (No. 2) [1990] Duty of confidentiality

A retired secret service employee sought to publish his memoirs from Australia. The British government sought to restrain publication there, and the defendants sought to report those proceedings, which would involve publication of the allegations made. The AG sought to restrain those publications.

Held: 'A duty of confidence arises when confidential information comes to the knowledge of a person (the confidant) in circumstances where he has notice, or is held to have agreed, that the information is confidential, with the effect that it would be just in all the circumstances that he should be precluded from disclosing the information to others'.

The law of Defamation, is relevant in cases where there is a breach of confidentiality over patient records are covered by the Defamation Act 1996 where there is a breach of confidentiality and trust. This is possible where a healthcare professional falsifies patient records. It is difficult for a service user to trust a healthcare professional who falsifies records. Compensatory damages may be awarded to the patient by the court.

Box 4.5 Case: Kent v. Griffiths and others (2000) 3 CLL Rep 98

In a case where a challenge to the ambulance crew records resulted in the paramedics being found to have falsified their records to reflect that they responded to a patient call within nine minutes. Detailed examination of these and other records demonstrated that the time from call to arrival at the patient home had in fact been 30 minutes. Action against the paramedics then followed.

www.advancedpractice.scot.ns.uk/legal-and-ethics-guidance/documentation-and-record-keeping/contemporaneous-notes.aspx

The courts recognize the importance of accurate documentation and the end result is exemplified by the following case where communication is not evidenced through communication. Poor communication may result in errors with safety implications and patients being harmed. The following case is in point.

Box 4.6 Case: Gauntlett v Northampton HA [1985]

Gauntlett v Northampton HA [1985] is a case in which a service user in a mental health facility was known to be at risk of self-harm via setting herself on fire. Her visiting husband handed over a box of matches to the nurses as she had asked him to state the following, 'Take these because I'll set fire to myself'. He, in turn, handed the matches to the charge nurse, who failed to record or communicate the concern. Consequently, the patient was not monitored, and four days later, she set fire to the tee shirt she was wearing, resulting in extensive burns.

The courts may take a dim view in cases where notes are not documented accurately and contemporaneously. They may also take the view that if it is not written, it did not happen. If there is accurate record-keeping, then in all probability, this will be relied upon as a record of events and, in the following case, obtaining consent. When information is not written down, people may forget or choose to invent something else at a later date.

Box 4.7 Case: McLennan v Newcastle HA [1992] 3 Med LR

This case provides a certain amount of legal weight to record-keeping. In this case a patient alleged that she had not been told of the relatively high risks in connection to her operation. The surgeon, however, had written in her notes that the risks were disclosed and understood by the patient, and consequently the judge decided that in all probability the patient had indeed been told of the risks. Note: the written entry was dated at the time of discussions with the patient

In the event of a request for records with a view to complain or litigate, the Data Protection Act 1998 provides for service users to have access to their records, both paper-based and computer-held. The Freedom of Information Act 2003, 2014 allows rights of access to anyone, all information which is not covered by the Data Protection Act 1998. The Access to Health Records Act 1990 applies when access to records of a deceased person may be required for lodging complaints or litigation.

Information technology, artificial intelligence (AI)

This section will consider information, technology, and the relationship between human technology and artificial intelligence (AI) in respect of diagnosis, treatment and rehabilitation of patients.

> Artificial intelligence (AI), the ability of a digital computer or computer-controlled robot to perform tasks commonly associated with intelligent beings. The term is frequently applied to the project of developing systems endowed with the intellectual processes characteristic of humans, such as the ability to reason, discover meaning, generalize, or learn from past experience. Since the development of the digital computer in the 1940s, it has been demonstrated that computers can be programmed to carry out very complex tasks—as, for example, discovering proofs for mathematical theorems.
> BRITANNICAhttps://www.britannica.com/technology/artificial-intelligence

Patient records and data is now mostly stored on a computer database subject to the Computer Misuse Act 1990 requires secure storage of such information. There is nowadays a link to regional or national systems the streams of data, One example is information access for ambulance paramedics. National or regional research may inform policy makers on epidemiology and underlying trends. Without technology it would not be possible to report on this or to share information. According to the NHS Digital's deputy chief executive, 'The NHS is living "in the dark ages" when it comes to technology, while outpatient services "would still be recognised" by Victorian doctors according to health tech leaders' (Rapson J [2019]).

Confidential information related to patient care is nowadays mostly stored on computer databases with limited paper copies. How safe are these IT systems? There is demonstrably the risk of this information not being 100 per cent secure enough with always a possibility that the information security systems may be breached. Exceptions may arise, as discussed above, under the common law on how these bases may be used by authorities, as where there is 'an overriding public interest' (DoH, 1999). It is therefore a challenge for IT database managers to ensure secure data system for patient related records.

Artificial Intelligence (AI) has also been defined as,

> ... the ability of a digital computer or computer-controlled robot to perform tasks commonly associated with intelligent beings. The term is frequently applied to the project of developing systems endowed with the intellectual processes characteristic of humans, such as the ability to reason, discover meaning, generalize, or learn from past experience AI has become more and more complex and sophisticated with an increased role of technology and should arguably improve the quality of investigations, early detection and diagnosis as well as treatment.
> (Copeland 2020)

AI has changed the nature of medical science and the relationship between human be-ings (healthcare professionals) and how they work with technology. It is clearly able to expedite investigations, confirm a more accurate diagnosis and enhance the treatment, thus improving outcomes. This is of course dependent on the patient's prognosis and response to treatment as well as, the knowledge and skills of the physician, and the appropriateness of the interventions implemented. There may be a treatment regime recommended by the algorithm, such as a course of medication or surgical procedures as well as interventions by other therapists to which a patient may or may not respond. AI may provide a degree of probability which has no guarantee to expected outcomes. Who is accountable if things go wrong; the IT manufacturer or the clinician and can the latter override the recommended course of treatment? Automated computer sys-tems may be breached by malicious software.

Ethical issues are inevitably raised regarding whether clinical judgement and decision-making should be left to computers or to humans and if so to what extent? The four principles of bioethics apply (Beauchamp and Childress, 2013). If a wrong decision or treatment option is chosen and implemented based on technology, is the liability with the doctor or the technologist who devised what turns out to have a faulty programme design? This is a whole new level of accountability. While technology has brought with it innovations and advantages, the reality is that it may be difficult to assess the level of 'harm' that technology and artificial intelligence may contribute during a patient treatment. This may create a headache for the courts in establishing liability and proportionate damages.

It is useful to consider briefly in what contexts artificial intelligence is used within health care. One positive example is an AI programme which is able to diagnose skin cancer more accurately than a fully qualified dermatologist (Esteva et al., 2017). The advance of medicine has been enhanced by AI through early diagnosis. Examples are monitoring, predicting disease prognosis through prescribing and prevention of ad-verse drug reaction, targeting prediabetic diagnosis and chronic disease management and identifying cancers (Bresnick, 2018). This may also be applicable to mental health treatment (Luxton, 2016).

A disadvantage of the use of AI, which raises questions on ethical considerations of the possibility of replacement of humans by computers and robotics, is that

> It's possible that the roles of radiologist, pathologist, and laboratory physician will cease to be separate in the future. Perhaps we will become total integrators of diagnostic information, working together more closely in integrated diagnostic departments to bring together all the pieces of the diagnostic puzzle as quickly as possible.
>
> (Bram Stieltjes 2019)

Unanswered questions remain about the real and perceived benefits as well as potential abuse of technology such as manipulation of the impulse settings of a neurostimulator implant inserted into the brain of a patient with Parkinson's disease. An example of incorrectly programmed radiation therapy could have disastrous consequences. What happens with the possibility of robots looking after vulnerable people with mobility problems? The issue lies with the design and programming of any device with an appli-cation or programme designed for certain actions. The transformation of the health-care provision through technology cannot be underestimated, though for service users no AI can take the place of humans. In spite of development in technology and AI, there may be an ethical case for more of the human touch (rather than less), though it could be argued that AI will give clinicians more time to show their patients that they care and for better treatment outcomes.

Conclusion

Ethical considerations and legal obligations are at the heart of healthcare provision and patient information. The NMC Code (2018) recognizes this. A healthcare professional owes a duty of care to the service user to ensure that they are not harmed by their negligent actions or omissions and this includes disclosure of confidential information.

Healthcare professionals have a duty of care to maintain accurate and quality records as this may affect care delivery and continuity of care, hence the need for accuracy.

Medical records may be used as evidence (in a court of law) of the care that has been given as well as communication between the patient and the nurse, the MDT and family members, this being one of the 6 C's. Clinical governance will consider the quality of records. Nurses owe the patient a duty of confidentiality requires the nurse to ensure security of all patient-identifiable information. Most of the data is now held on computer databases and this means that IT managers and all staff employed by healthcare providers have an obligation in common law as well as their employment contract, to ensure security of patient-identifiable information.

The introduction of AI in health care has been a game-changer and part and parcel of overall advances in modern medicine which should result in an improvement in patient outcomes. It is important to keep everything in perspective by acknowledging the benefits of improving the quality and timing of diagnosis, though without taking away the human element of healthcare professionals who use AI as a tool to complement rather than substitute their knowledge and skills of specialist medical staff through over-reliance on it. Ethical questions may arise in terms of substituting clinical decision-making with algorithms.

Freedom of Information (Scotland) Act 2002.

References

Access to Health Records Act 1990, s3(1) (f).

Adair J, Skills of Leadership, Surrey, Gower Publishing Ltd, 1984.

AG v Guardian Newspapers Ltd. (No. 2) [1990].

Beauchamp TL and Childress JF. *Principles of bio-medical ethics*, 7th ed. Oxford: Oxford University Press, 2013.

Bresnick J (2018) Artificial intelligence promises a new paradigm for healthcare investigations and diagnosis. Available online at: https://healthitanalytics.com/features/artificial-intelligence-promises-a-new-paradigm-for-healthcare.

Bram Stieltjes, MD, Head of Research Coordination at the Radiology and Nuclear Medicine Clinic at University Hospital Basel, Switzerland, *Algorithms: All Set to Shape Tomorrow's Medicine*, Medical Solutions, 2019.

Britannica, Artificial Intelligence definition. Available online at: https://www.britannica.com/technology/artificial-intelligence (accessed on 18th April 2020).

Buka P, Davis M, Pereira M (2016) Care of Vulnerable Older People, Basingstoke, Macmillan Press.

Caldicott Committee. *Report on the review of patient-identifiable information.* London: Department of Health, 1997.

Computer Misuse Act 1990.

Copeland B J at the University of Canterbury, Encyclopaedia Britannica (2020) Available online at: https://www.britannica.com/technology/artificial-intelligence (accessed on 30th October 2019).

Criminal Appeal Act 1995.

Data Protection Act 1998 implementing UK law European Directive 95/46/EC on the processing of personal data. Available online at: https://www.gov.uk/data-protection/the-data-protection-act (accessed on 1st July 2019).

Data Protection Act 1998, Schedule 2. 3.

Data Protection Act, General Data Protection Regulation (GDPR) 2018.

Defamation Acts 1996 and 2013.

Department of Health (2003) Confidentiality NHS Code of practice. Available online at: https://assets.publishing.service.gov.uk/government/uploads/system/uploads/attachment_data/file/200146/Confidentiality_-_NHS_Code_of_Practice.pdf (accessed on 21st December 2019).

DoH (1999) Health Service Circular: HSC 1999/012.

Donoghue v Stevenson, [1932] UKHL 100 AC 562 (HL).

Esteva A, Kuprel B, Novoa R A, et al. Dermatologist-level classification of skin with deep cancer neural networks. *Nature* 2017; 542(7639): 115–8. Available online at: View Article Pub Med Google Scholar (accessed on 20th June 2019).

Freedom of Information Act 2003, 2014.

Freedom of Information (Scotland) Act 2002.

Gauntlett v Northampton HA [1985].

Government of Wales Act 1998.

Health and Social Care Act 2001, s60.

Human Rights Act 1998, Art 8.

Information Commissioner's Offices (2013) Available online at: http://www.ico.gov.uk/what_we_cover/data_protection/legislation_in_full.aspx (accessed on 1st July 2019).

Kent v. Griffiths and others (2000) 3 CLL Rep 98.

Luxton DD. *Artificial intelligence in behavioral and mental health care.* San Diego: Elsevier Academic Press, 2016.

McLennan v Newcastle HA [1992] 3 Med LR.

Miller & Another v Health Service Commissioner for England [2018] EWCA Civ 144.

NHS Act 2006.

NMC (2009) Record keeping Guidance for nurses and midwives. Available online at: https://nipec.hscni.net/download/projects/previous_work/highstandards_education/improving_recordkeeping/publications/nmcGuidanceRecordKeepingGuidanceforNursesandMidwives.pdf. (accessed on 18th April 2020).

NMC (2015) Guidance for nurses and midwives on record keeping [Online]. Available online at: https://www.google.co.uk/webhp?source=search_app&gfe_rd=cr&ei=PLPIVoifMO_S8Ae6mqiABw&gws_rd=ssl#q=nmc+record+keeping+guidance+ (accessed on 12th February 2018).

NMC Code (2018) Professional standards of practice and behaviour for nurses and midwives and nursing associates. Available online at: https://www.nmc.org.uk/globalassets/site documents/nmc-publications/revised-new-nmc-code (accessed on 2nd February 2018).

Police and Criminal Evidence Act (PACE) 1984.

Public Health (Control of Disease) Act 1984.

Public Records Act 1958, s 3.

Public Records Act (Northern Ireland) 1923.

Public Records (Scotland) Act 1937.

Rapson J (2019) NHS living in the 'dark ages'. Available online at: https://www.hsj.co.uk/nhs-digital-hscic/15219.subject (accessed on 22nd June 2019).

RCN (2017) Record keeping, the facts. Available online at: https://www.rcn.org.uk/professional-development/publications/pub-006051 (accessed on 21st December 2019).

Road Traffic Act 1988.

Shiraishi J, Li Q, Appelbaum D, Doi K (2011) Computer-aided diagnosis and artificial intelligence in clinical imaging. *Seminars in Nuclear Medicine* November 2011; 41(6): 449–2. Available online at: https://www.sciencedirect.com/science/article/abs/pii/S0001299811000742?via%-3Dihub (accessed on 20th April 2020).

Consent to treatment, patient autonomy

Chapter outline

Introduction

This chapter considers the nature of consent as well as exceptions such as when a patient is deemed to lack consent. What happens in cases where a patient lacks mental capacity, and can necessity ever be justified as a valid defence for healthcare professionals who may be challenged for breach of human rights (Human Rights Act 1998, Article 3)? What are the requirements for consent to be valid? This raises some ethical and moral issues not only about the patient's autonomy but also about the expected impact of beneficence and nonmaleficence of nursing actions, which includes ensuring that consent is properly obtained. All patients should always be presumed to have the competence/mental capacity (related to cognition) to choose – until established otherwise (Mental Capacity Act 2005). Consent should normally be obtained or alternatively where a patient lacks capacity, act in their best interest and within a relevant legal framework. One example is detaining a client under the Mental Health Act 1983.

What is consent?

The concept of consent goes to the heart of ethics and the issues of human freedom and autonomy to make decisions. This includes the ability to make informed choices about our lives as well as any necessary treatment. A patient receiving care may be in a vulnerable position if their judgement is impaired in some way. This means that there should be no presumption that blanket consent to all forms of treatment is presumed once the patient is receiving treatment. It is therefore an important aspect of communication that, in normal circumstances, the nurse needs to ensure that the patient has consented before any treatment is provided (Nursing and Midwifery Council [NMC], 2018). One example is before invasive procedures such as inserting a nasogastric tube or administering an enema to a patient.

Because of fundamental human rights, a client does not depend on 'paternalism' to make a choice on treatment options. Principlism and the ethical basis of treatment mean that under the principle of beneficence, any treatment provided should benefit the patient; the converse is maltreatment with the need to avoid futile treatment as this could be non-maleficence, that is, avoiding harm (Beauchamp and Childress, 2013). All clients should receive fair treatment, and their right to choose a course of action falls under the principle of autonomy (Beauchamp and Childress, 2013). Patient autonomy is linked to capacity, and they are entitled to make an informed choice (Article 8 of the Human Rights Act 1998). The nurse should be guided by a framework of consent (NMC, Code 2018), as found in the national guidelines as well as local protocol. Some of the key questions they should contemplate are:

1. Which category of clients should have the right to consent?
2. How should life-threatening emergency situations be addressed when there may not be an opportunity to obtain consent?
3. What should happen when the client lacks consent?
4. Are there circumstances when consent may be overridden without breaching the client's rights?

For consent to be valid, it must be voluntary and informed, and the person consenting must have the capacity to make the decision. This means that:

- voluntary – the decision to either consent or not to consent to treatment must be made by the person, and must not be influenced by pressure from medical staff, friends or family
- informed – the person must be given all of the information about what the treatment involves, including the benefits and risks, whether there are reasonable alternative treatments, and what will happen if treatment does not go ahead
- capacity – the person must be capable of giving consent, which means they understand the information given to them and can use it to make an informed decision
  (NHS https://www.nhs.uk/conditions/consent-to-treatment/)

Box 5.1 Thinking point

A patient is admitted for day-stay surgery for a minor gynaecological procedure. This is, however, carried out under a general anaesthetic. Consider the role of the nurse in relation to consent.

1   What are the ethical and legal considerations for obtaining 'informed' consent?
2   What tools for determining mental capacity are in use in your workplace?

Exerting any pressure or undue influence is grounds for invalidating that consent (Doyal, 2002). Consent may be classified as,

- Expressed (or express) – written or oral,
- Implicit – implied or tacit,

- General,
- Specific.

Expressed (or express) consent

This type of consent involves a clear expression by the patient of their wishes. Expressed or express consent must be explicit, or obvious and the patient must be given the opportunity to openly express their agreement to the operation or examination and this may be either written or verbal.

> Consent is often wrongly equated with a patient's signature on a consent form. A signature on a form is evidence that the patient has given consent but is not proof of valid consent. If a patient is rushed into signing a form, on the basis of too little information, the consent may not be valid, despite the signature. Similarly, if a patient has given valid verbal consent, the fact that they are physically unable to sign the form is no bar to treatment. Patients may, if they wish, withdraw consent after they have signed a form: the signature is evidence of the process of consent-giving, not a binding contract.
>
> (Department of Health, 2001a, updated in 2009)

Consent may be written or verbal. Both forms of consent are valid, although for evidence it is obviously easier to establish for consent if this is in writing as it may be difficult to establish verbal consent. In time person may have a different recollection of events, for whatever reason. The use of a witness would be the only way of establishing this, should evidence of past consent need to be proved in a court of law. Problems may arise as a witness may forget the events, their recollection of events may change, they may move away to another job or they may have died by the time a case comes to court. There is, in fact, no legal requirement for expressed consent to be in writing as the patient may be unable to write but have the capacity to consent. If a patient is witnessed writing a mark such as an 'x' on the consent form, how easy or difficult is it to ascribe that signature to them at a later date.

For the consent to be valid, the patient must

- be competent to take the particular decision;
- have received sufficient information to take it;
- not be acting under duress.

(Department of Health, 2001a, updated in 2009)

Implicit or tacit consent

The presence of consent can also be established by inference of the conduct of the patient, although there may be difficulties in establishing this in retrospect. The term 'implicit' is more closely aligned to treatment, while 'tacit' is used in a much wider sense and is broadly applied by moral philosophers such as Locke (Nozick, 1974). This type of consent is sometimes called 'tacit' as the patient does not need to express this verbally; only their actions are required. This may also be open to abuse if treatment is provided on the erroneous assumption that the patient has given permission for treatment or examination; hence, it is important that the nurse establish the fact that a patient is happy for a treatment intervention to go ahead.

Box 5.2 Case: Beatty v Cullingworth Q.B. Unreported [1896] 44 CENT. L.J. 153 (s896)

The patient (who was a nurse) consented to removal of her right ovary, specifically telling the surgeon beforehand that if both ovaries were found to be diseased, neither should be removed. The surgeon said that she should leave that to him, to which she made no reply. At operation, both ovaries were removed as the left as well as the right was found to be diseased. When the case came to trial, the judge said, 'if a medical man undertook an operation, it was a humane thing for him to do everything in his power to remove the mischief'. The jury returned a verdict for the defendant (the surgeon), despite the absence of consent.

An example of implied consent is where a patient is approached by a nurse with a syringe injection and they offer their hand as a sign that they agree to the procedure being carried out. Compare and contrast the above case with the American case below (which is only persuasive and not binding in the UK courts), which illustrates this point.

Box 5.3 Case: O'Brien v Cunard SS Co. [1891] 28 NE 266

In this case an individual (on the defendant's ship) had stood in the queue and offered her arm for vaccination, and then subsequently testified that she did not wish to be vaccinated and had not given her consent. The courts held that there was implied consent – by willingly standing in the queue and offering her arm, and accordingly in a similar instance treatment would be justified.

A similar defence for a clinician may be allowed in court if they acted in the belief that the patient had been able to give consent by actively taking steps in acceptance of any treatment offered. The courts would also accept the use of reasonable intervening actions, which would be supported by the *Bolam* standards of practice (see Chapter 1, 'Concept of Law and Human Rights').

Blanket consent

This section considers the effectiveness of 'blanket' agreements for treatment to go ahead. The danger is that this may be open to challenge should the patient be given treatment without understanding it, or under false pretences. Although this sounds valid from a contractual point of view, there is the possibility of abuse with the patient's rights being overridden under Article 3 of Human Rights Act (HRA) 1998. It is, however, useful in a laparoscopy-type operation where the surgeon has the option to pursue either an alternative course of action or a more extensive operation should the outcome turn out to be different from that expected, as shown in the following case. It is possible that in the course of an exploratory operation a surgeon may find a condition other than the one he expected, which requires a more extensive operation. The patient should be warned of this possibility so that they may give consent prior to surgery. The implication of giving blanket consent is that clinicians cannot give any guarantee that the patient's rights will be ensured. In ordinary circumstances, informed consent must be obtained before any treatment. Exceptions to the rule are clearly laid out in Department of Health (2001a) guidelines.

Specific consent

Any consent given by a patient must be related to the specific treatment or procedure without the discretion of the nurse to choose a completely different alternative, which may not have been agreed to by the patient.

The following case is authority for the view that a patient should be informed of the nature and extent of the proposed treatment or surgery and not only the benefits but also the risks.

Box 5.4 Case: Williamson v East London and City Health Authority, HA [1998], Lloyds Reports, Med 6, [1990]

The plaintiff had previously been given silicone gel breast implants at the age of 30 for cosmetic reasons and subsequently developed multiple lumps, which the surgeon associated with a leak from the silicone implant. The plaintiff, having consented to breast surgery silicone replacement and lump excision only, was instead given a more radical operation. Having developed multiple lumps, a radical mastectomy operation was performed, without her consent. The court found that there had been no prior explanation by the surgeon and that the patient had not consented to the extensive surgery. she was awarded damages of £20,000 for pain and suffering as a result of the 'negligent' action in failing to obtain consent to the operation performed.

Human rights and patient autonomy

Patient autonomy is reinforced by the Montgomery Case, that 'the doctor [is] under a duty to inform the patient of the material risks inherent in the treatment. A risk [is] material, for these purposes, if a reasonably prudent patient in the situation of the patient would think it significant' (Lord Scarman, Para 47, *Montgomery v Lanarkshire Health Board [2015] UKSC 11*). The concept of paternalism has been at the centre of traditional medicine and nursing, with the patient being a small player and not questioning clinical judgements being on the receiving end. However, difficulties and ethical issues arise when doctors and nurses start to impose their own values on others who may not share those (Campbell et al., 2001). The general public is now more aware of their rights and has access to information from sources such as the media and the Internet. More recently, Article 8(1) of the HRA 1998 asserts that 'everyone has the right to respect for his private and family life, his home and his correspondence'. This article gives individuals some 'moral autonomy' (Hoffman and Rowe, 2013). Thus, for the nurse, safeguarding the patient's autonomy and their entitlement to self-determination through consent to treatment is important. There are, however, exceptions, for example, in infectious disease control, where maintaining privacy may be putting the public at risk (Public Health [Control of Diseases] Act 1984, as amended by the Health and Social Care Act 2008).

In a treatment setting 'informed' refers to the choice of useful therapies, usefulness being a professional decision. The informing process needs a good relationship between patient and doctor. In a research setting the principles are also generally agreed: The risks must not be disproportionate; and the patient (or guardian in some psychiatric settings) has to give informed consent. The first applies also where consent is not possible but here, determinations of risks and of benefits to self and others have to have the protection of the law.

(WHO, 2003)

In a therapeutic relationship, the patient has a right to have informed consent prior to treatment. This means that a sufficient degree of information must be given to allow them to make a balanced judgement as to whether to accept treatment or not. The role of the nurse should be to facilitate this process for the patient by empowering them to make decisions affecting their treatment. It is possible that a patient may not wish to receive such information, but nevertheless, the nurse must provide the patient with that opportunity to seek any clarification for treatment and the opportunity to give consent or to decline treatment.

The issue of autonomy has been at the heart of the debate for philosophers such as Immanuel Kant (1724–1804), who recognized that people have a natural right to choose because they are born with a free will (the categorical imperative), with the assumption that this comes with their ability to make a rational judgement. Others, such as John Stuart Mill (1806–73), have, however, suggested that autonomy is a natural human freedom of the expression of one's opinion as well as to live in a way that expresses 'individuality' (Mill, 1993). The ethical basis of autonomy is the right to 'respect' a person's right to self-determination (Blackburn, 2001). This principle is applicable to the treatment environment, that is, allowing the patient to choose treatment, and this was recognized in law in the following landmark case.

Box 5.5 Case: Schloendorff v Society of New York Hospital 211 NY; 105 NE 92, 93 [1914]; 106 NE 93; NY [1914]

A woman had consented to an abdominal examination under anaesthesia but not to a surgical operation. Knowing this to be the case the surgeon went ahead to operate and remove a tumour. The patient sued for battery. Justice Cardozo's opinion (p. 304) expressed what has now become the foundation for the concept of informed consent and for an individual patient's right of autonomy and self-determination: 'every human being of adult years and sound mind has a right to determine what shall be done with his own body; and a surgeon who performs an operation without his patient's consent commits an assault for which he is liable in damages'.

Patient autonomy and mental capacity

Autonomy is a basic human right in both ethics and law, and this is central to consent as human beings have the capacity to weigh the information before them and deliberate or make a considered choice (Furrow, 2005). Following the above legal principle, autonomy is also the ability or capacity to weigh the options and then choose moral alternatives (Thompson et al., 2006). The patient has a basic human right to autonomy, which is defined in law. If this right is infringed, it is therefore the patient's prerogative to choose to accept or to decline treatment, knowing that the consequences may be detrimental to their health. For the injured party (the patient), infringement of such a right may give rise to an action for damages in tort against another person who is alleged to have violated that right (Fletcher and Buka, 1999). This right is, nevertheless, not absolute, and it is for the courts to define based on the statutory provisions as interpreted in pre-existing case law. There is also a presumption in law that all adults are competent unless proven otherwise. For individuals who are competent the patient's right to decline treatment regardless of the possible adverse outcome is recognized in common law as illustrated in the *St George's Healthcare National Health Service Trust v S* (no. 2) reported in *The Times* Law Report of 3 August 1998. A patient also has the right to withdraw any previously given and obtained consent.

The Mental Capacity Act 2005 (MCA, 2005) came into force from April 2007, thus empowering patients and strengthening current rules. The equivalent Scottish statute is the Adults with Incapacity (Scotland) Act 2000. Under the MCA 2005 the guiding principles for determining capacity are

(1) The following principles apply for the purposes of this Act.
(2) A person must be assumed to have capacity unless it is established that he lacks capacity.
(3) A person is not to be treated as unable to make a decision unless all practicable steps to help him to do so have been taken without success.
(4) A person is not to be treated as unable to make a decision merely because he makes an unwise decision.
(5) An act done or decision made, under this Act for or on behalf of a person who lacks capacity must be done, or made, in his best interests.
(6) Before the act is done, or the decision is made, regard must be had to whether the purpose for which it is needed can be as effectively achieved in a way that is less restrictive of the person's rights and freedom of action.

(Section 1 of MCA 2005)

Box 5.6 Thinking point

Mrs X is a frail 70-year-old widow who was first diagnosed with multiple sclerosis 20 years ago, though getting progressively worse) and has developed mild Dementia has increasingly become dependent on two regular carers for personal care. She has occasional urinal incontinent and needs helps with washing and dressing, requiring care twice a day. Her son, who lives abroad, suspects that her friend and trusted informal carer has been regularly withdrawing large sums of money without Mrs X's consent and she does not always provide receipts for shopping. Mrs X suspects this but is afraid to challenge her and say anything in case she loses her, unbeknown to them the carer has a criminal record but has managed to get this job through an agency, which failed to check her credentials on engaging her.
What advice would you give to Mrs X's son?

The Mental Capacity Act (MCA) 2005 is applicable on assessment of a person's capacity, which should be based on a 'decision-specific' test.

- A presumption of capacity – every adult has the right to make his or her own decisions and must be assumed to have capacity to do so unless it is proved otherwise.
- The right for individuals to be supported to make their own decisions – people must be given all appropriate help before anyone concludes that they cannot make their own decisions.

- That individuals must retain the right to make what might be seen as eccentric or unwise decision.
- Best interests – anything done for or on behalf of people without capacity must be in their best interest.
- Least restrictive intervention – anything done for or on behalf of people without capacity should be the least restrictive of their basic rights and freedoms.
(Section 1 of Mental Capacity Act 2005)

There is now no presumption of incapacity based on a patient's medical condition or state of mind (Section 2 of MCA 2005). During any decision-making process, where a service user lacks capacity their 'best interests' must be at the centre. The above principles are seen as key to providing new safeguards for people lacking in capacity. In July 2018, a Mental Capacity Amendment Bill was passed, and this means that this has been law since May 2019. It replaces the Deprivation of Liberty Safeguards (DoLS) with a scheme known as the Liberty Protection Safeguards.

One example of protection of the vulnerable patient (who lacks capacity) based on Scots law is the Mental Health (Care and Treatment) (Scotland) Act 2003. Guardianship is addressed in Chapter 5, Section 7, which states that the guardian, and only the guardian herself or himself, has the power to;

- require the person to live at a particular place,
- require the person to go to specific places at specific times for the purpose of medical treatment.

This is nevertheless subject to:

2) The functions of the judge under this Part of this Act shall be exercisable where, after considering medical evidence, he is satisfied that a person is incapable, by reason of mental disorder, of managing and administering his property and affairs; and a person as to whom the judge is so satisfied is referred to in this Part of this Act as a patient.
(Section 94(2) of the Mental Health Act 1983)

This section would also allow a judge to make a ruling regarding administration of such a patient's property under Section 95 of the same statute.

Section 46 of the MCA 2005 introduced new provisions for the Court of Protection, giving special wider powers to the Court of Protection for deciding on matters related to a patient's incapacity. In Scotland the Adults with Incapacity (Scotland) Act (2008) applies. In the same vein, the Mental Health Act 2007 aims to redefine treatment of those who need treatment while improving the safeguarding of individuals who lack capacity, for example, involuntary commitment, only if 'appropriate treatment' is available. This statute also provides for healthcare advocates or proxies (Scotland) and for supervised community treatment. This provides the power for a supervised discharge with power to return a non-compliant patient to a hospital for compulsory treatment.

For those with mental capacity, they may choose to appoint a financial 'advocate' to manage their affairs when they lack the capacity to choose. There are two main categories: ordinary power of attorney and lasting power of attorney.

Ordinary power of attorney

In this category, a person may choose any person whom they so wish to represent them. When the patient loses their capacity for decision-making, a representative to whom such power is delegated subsequently has the power to make decisions on their behalf. In law, there is a presumption that any decisions they make will be in the best interests of the person they represent. In addition, the person who delegates this power may revoke this power at any time.

lasting power of attorney.

A solicitor is normally required for verifying the wishes of the person drawing up a legal deed and their capacity to do so. A person chosen to manage their financial affairs will have the right to carry out any necessary transactions should the person drawing up the deed lose their mental capacity. The physical or mental incapacity may be due to illness.

Court of Protection (sections 93–98 of Mental Health act 1983) is required for individuals who lack mental capacity and is the most appropriate route for safeguarding their interests. An application to the court must be supported by consultant medical opinion in the relevant documents of the patient's state of mind. If the court accepts this, it appoints a 'receiver' who is answerable to the court. One way of safeguarding the interests of a vulnerable person is the requirement for accounts to be submitted to the court periodically. The Court of Protection is, nevertheless, not without criticism and can be 'archaic, bureaucratic'. This is evident from the number of cases which go to the court where a single judge deliberates and decides.

The right to choose to accept or decline treatment, based on an informed choice, is based on Article 8 of the Human Rights Act 1998, defined as

> The rights to respect for private and family life,
> 1. Everyone has the right to respect for his private and family life, his home and his correspondence.

The Mental Capacity Act 2005 defines the nature of consent, and competence is specific to consent, even if the client lacks mental capacity in other aspects or, indeed, at other times. The relationship between the nurse and their patient is based on trust and a need for purposeful and effective communication by making sure you gain consent prior to treatment and 'uphold people's rights to be fully involved in decisions about their care' and are required to be aware of the law on mental capacity (NMC, 2018). As part of this communication process it is normal that most patients may wish to ask questions related to their treatment. The nurse has a moral and legal duty to ensure that the patient's autonomy is respected. This may, however, not be applicable when a patient lacks capacity. In addition, other ethical principles such as beneficence require the promotion of good, while non-maleficence focusses on avoiding any action which may be detrimental to the patient's health (by denying them their freedom of choice) and within Bioethical framework (Beauchamp and Childress, 2013). The guidelines are clear about the clinician's responsibility for obtaining consent and for empowering the patient. It is possible for a specially trained member of the multi-disciplinary team, who is not carrying out the procedure, to obtain consent from the patient:

1. The health professional carrying out the procedure is ultimately responsible for ensuring that the patient is genuinely consenting to what is being done: it is they who will be held responsible in law if this is challenged later.
2. Where oral or non-verbal consent is being sought at the point the procedure is carried out, this will naturally be done by the health professional responsible. However, teamwork is a crucial part of the way the NHS operates, and where written consent is being sought it may be appropriate for other members of the team to participate in the process of seeking consent.

(Department of Health, 2001b)

Where there is lack of consent there is the possibility of litigation for negligence and civil actions for trespass to the person (including assault and battery). Assault is putting another person in a state of fear for their safety, and battery involves unwanted physical contact. Carrying out procedures without consent may amount to battery or assault. Where a patient is detained in hospital against their wishes this may amount to false imprisonment unless the Mental Health Act 1983 is applied. Assault and battery may be subject to criminal prosecution under the Offences against the Person Act 1861 and other statutes.

To be able to provide adequate information, the clinician should be capable of performing or understanding the nature of the procedure which the patient will undergo. The patient should be given a sufficient degree of information, options and the related benefits and any risks involved. For instance, where a surgical operation is concerned, the law expects a surgeon to inform the patient about the benefits and risks of a procedure. In order to enable patients to make an informed choice the standard of care is decided by the *Bolam* case, 'standard of a reasonable skilled person who professes to have those skills', and the law will judge a professional by the standard of a 'reasonable' nurse.

It is acknowledged that the patient has a right to refuse treatment, though updated by the NMC Code (2018), and earlier medical guidelines illustrated the patient's right to refuse treatment.

> You must respect any refusal of treatment given when the patient was competent, provided the decision in the advance statement is clearly applicable to the present circumstances, and there is no reason to believe that the patient has changed his/ her mind. Where an advance statement of this kind is not available, the patient's known wishes should be taken into account.
>
> (GMC, 1999)

A clinician must always look to their own professional code of conduct as well as to local policies and guidelines for guidance. The patient must be given a sufficient degree of information to enable them to make an informed choice about whether to consent to the treatment or procedure. A doctor does not have to disclose all the risks (Giliker and Bethwith, 2011). The *Bolam* principle was applied in the case of *Sidaway v Board of Governors of the Bethlem Royal Hospital and the Maudsley Hospital* [1985] AC 871, where the plaintiff had a chronic neck condition and the surgeon recommended an operation. The surgeon failed to warn the patient of a small risk (1 per cent), as the operation was within less than 3 cm of the spinal cord. The outcome of the operation resulted in severing of the spine, causing paralysis. The patient said that she would not have agreed to the operation had she known the risk. The House of Lords *held* that as the risk was minimal, autonomy was not absolute and that the patient is not always the best judge on the level of information to be given. On the basis of this case it could be argued that in this instance it was effectively accepted that sometimes paternalism might be justifiable. In contrast, the case of *Chester v Ashfar* [2004] UKHL 41 (below) went the other way, adopting a patient-focussed approach, which affirmed the patient's right to be informed of any avoidable risk, no matter how minor.

Box 5.7 Case: Chester v Ashfar [2004] UKHL 41

A surgeon performing a Caesarean section discovered fibroid tumours. Due to his concern about the risk posed by a second pregnancy he went ahead and sterilized the patient. The patient went to court seeking damages on the grounds that she had not consented to the operation.

Held: The doctor was liable. And furthermore, while the first operation was required, the sterilization was convenient at the time as there was no evidence that the fibroids posed an immediate danger to the patient's life or health. Informed consent and capacity were set out based on Dr Easterman's expert evidence with the decision-making process in three stages, with Thorpe setting out a three-tier test:

whether the patient comprehended and retained information,
whether they believed it,
whether they could weigh in the balance and arrive at a choice.

Box 5.8 Thinking point

Mrs X, aged 80, lives on her own and is normally independent, apart from having home help twice weekly. She suffers from mild dementia but has reasonable awareness of what is going on. She has one son who visits weekly with his own family. She has been admitted to A&E following a fall, and the X-rays have confirmed a fractured neck of femur, requiring surgery. The surgeons are concerned that on admission Mrs X is very confused and unable to understand relevant information or give informed consent.

What are the current guidelines for managing individuals who lack mental capacity to consent, before surgery can be undertaken?

If Mrs X has a 'living will' with advance directives in her medical records, how would this affect her consent to treatment?

The law today is interpreted in the Montgomery Case 2015 (a Supreme Court case identified above, in this chapter). As a professional, the nurse has a duty to protect their patient's right to autonomy. For patients who are incompetent or lack capacity there is an expectation that nurses will advocate for these patients.

Legal scholars such as Hart (1968, p. 5) recognize that informed consent is part of human freedom but, nevertheless, is not absolute as 'there may be grounds justifying the legal coercion of the individual other than the prevention of harm to others'. UK law recognizes the clearly defined right of a patient not to be given treatment against his or her will, and not to be treated in the complete absence of consent. However, in interpretation of the law, judges in the UK have not developed a full doctrine of 'informed consent'. Lord Donaldson has subsequently set out the UK position as follows:

Box 5.9 Case: Re T [1992] 9 BMLR 46

Court of Appeal, Civil Division, denied an appeal on behalf of a critically ill, unconscious woman who had been given a blood transfusion upon court order after having previously refused to consent to one. The woman's mother, a Jehovah's Witness, had apparently influenced the decision of the daughter, who was not a Jehovah's Witness. The Court of Appeal held that, though every adult has the right and capacity to refuse medical treatment, this presumption of capacity can be overridden upon a determination that factors such as confusion, unconsciousness, fatigue, or shock

(continued)

(continued)

> affect the patient's decision. When a patient refuses treatment, doctors must consider the importance of the treatment, and whether the patient's capacity was reduced. Doctors must also consider whether the patient's decision was made independently. Doctors who are faced with a patient's refusal of treatment in a life-threatening situation such as this should utilize the court system for assistance.
>
> https://www.ncbi.nlm.nih.gov/pubmed/11648226

For patients who lack capacity there are provisions in the Mental Capacity Act 2005 (Adults with Incapacity (Scotland) Act 2000). The advocate or 'deputy' is a person over the age of 18 who is appointed by the court. Under Section 20 of the Mental Capacity Act 2005, the deputy has limited powers and may not substitute the patient's decisions if they believe that the patient has the power to make that decision. For example, they may only decline treatment but may not demand treatment. Doctors may treat a patient based on their own clinical judgements. Those who lack capacity are defined as follows:

(1) For the purposes of this Act, a person lacks capacity in relation to a matter if at the material time he is unable to make a decision for himself in relation to the matter because of an impairment of, or a disturbance in the functioning of, the mind or brain.

If the lack of capacity is transient, due to an underlying medical condition, an infection, medication or disorientation, the nurse should consider obtaining consent another time, when the patient's capacity is evident (Section 4(2)). This may be difficult in practice if a patient suffers from spells of confusion. Individuals diagnosed with states of confusion, such as dementia, or with mental health conditions, such as schizophrenia, must be presumed to have the capacity to consent until and unless proven otherwise.

In order to determine whether a patient has the necessary capacity, the test adopted is that in *Re C Test/Re C Advice: Refusal of Treatment* [1994] 1 WLR 290. At times it is possible that a patient's 'best interests' should be considered due to a patient's lack of capacity only after consideration of the following:

(3) He must consider (a) whether it is likely that the person will at some time have capacity in relation to the matter in question, and (b) if it appears likely that he will, when that is likely to be.

(4) He must, so far as reasonably practicable, permit and encourage the person to participate, or to improve his ability to participate, as fully as possible in any act done for him and any decision affecting him.

(Section 4 of Mental Capacity Act 2005)

Box 5.10 Thinking point

J. is a 31-year-old service user who lives on his own, with no known next of kin, and he has been recently diagnosed with bipolar illness and was admitted as an emergency following violent conduct at home. He was detained under the Mental Health Act 1983, following a suicide attempt. On discharge, he claims that he had been 'assaulted' and restrained and given injection medications against his will.

Consider the appropriate sections of the mental Health Act 1983 which may affect him and identify the service user's human rights in this case.

Patients with mental health needs may be detained under Sections 2–5 of the Mental Health Act 1983 and be subject to compulsory treatment for the mental health condition under Section 63 of the Mental Health Act 1983, in urgent cases. However, *F v West Berkshire Health Authority and Another (Mental Health Act Commission Intervening)* [1989] 2 All ER at 545 shows that under Section 93(1)b of the same act, managing 'the affairs of patients' (limited to business affairs) did not extend to questions relating to the medical treatment of a patient. The court had therefore no jurisdiction to override such a patient's wishes on medical treatment. Part IV of MHA 1983 (i.e. Sections 56–64) applies only to medical treatment for mental disorder (i.e. psychiatric treatment).

In emergency situations, treatment may be given without seeking the patient's permission. The justification of such intervention is to preserve or save life. A doctor may not be prosecuted for trespass in emergency circumstances provided they can show that in so doing they were acting in the best interests of the patient. In situations dealing with those who lack mental capacity, either temporarily or permanently, decisions may also be made in the patient's best interests, but there is a danger, prompting the need for clear guidelines. When applied, the best interests principle, Section 4 of Mental Capacity Act 2005, should also take the following facts into consideration:

> 1.14. If you are treating a patient who lacks capacity and who also has a mental disorder, you should be aware of how the mental health legislation across the UK interacts with the law on mental capacity. See the other sources of information at the end of this guidance.
>
> (General Medical Council, 2008)

There are exceptions under Article 5(e) of HRA 1998. There are also public health law provisions for obtaining consent and detention for people with an infectious disease. This is necessary due to some cases of life-threatening situations and where a patient has previously clearly identified (in living wills) their wishes to decline treatment as illustrated:

> It is established that the principle of self-determination requires that respect must be given to the wishes of the patient, so that if an adult patient of sound mind refuses, however unreasonably, to consent to treatment or care by which his life would or might be prolonged, the doctors responsible for his care must give effect to his wishes, even though they do not consider it to be in his best interests to do so.
>
> (Per Lord Goff at p. 864 C, Airedale NHS Trust v Bland [1993] AC 789)

In the event of an action for battery (subject to the Offences Against the Person Act 1861) being brought against a clinician, their justification would also be that they acted through necessity. 'Necessity' is a defence in an emergency situation where life-saving actions are taken in the patient's best interests (see below on capacity).

Consent and children

In the case of children, Section 1 of the Children Act 1989 states, *inter alia* – Latin for 'among other issues' – that the overriding factor is 'paramountcy' of the child's welfare; the child's best interest is also applicable to the treatment of children, as in 'the ascertainable wishes and feelings of the child (considered in light of his age and understanding)' and 'any harm the child has suffered or is at risk of suffering'. (For more detailed information see Chapter 3, 'Life at the beginning to adulthood'). *Gillick v West Norfolk and Wisbech*

Area Health Authority [1985] 3 All ER 492 is authority for the principle that in certain circumstances a child under the age of 16 years could give valid consent (for example, in the case of contraceptives) without the involvement or knowledge of parents. The test was whether the child had a sufficient degree of understanding of what was proposed (Fraser, formerly Gillick, competence). This test is about capacity, not merely the ability to make a choice. However, in *Re S [1994]* 2 FLR 1065, a Scottish case, a girl, aged 15, who needed regular transfusions due to thalassaemia refused transfusion on religious grounds. The court held that she lacked the Fraser Competence, and the Gillick Guidelines were applied due to the patient's lack of understanding or full appreciation of the implication of not having a blood transfusion for a child under the age of 16. For children, however, parental consent cannot override a refusal of consent by a competent child who has the legal capacity to consent to his or her own treatment. The position is also clarified in Scots law: 'In the opinion of the qualified medical practitioner attending to him/her, he/she is capable of understanding the nature and the possible consequences of the procedure or treatment', under Section 2(4) of the Legal Capacity (Scotland) Act 1991.

Parents or those with parental responsibility are normally expected by the law to make decisions on behalf of their children under the age of 18 in England or 16 in Scotland, unless the child has the capacity under the 'Fraser Competence'. Difficulties may arise for the nurse if there is conflict between the wishes of the parents and those of the child. Parents may not override a competent minor's decision. There is sometimes a need for a judicial review under the inherent *parens patriae* (Latin), literally 'father of the country' (which is the jurisdiction of the court, which may be exercised by the High Court, Family Division), with the aim of making the child a ward of the court. The role of the courts is highlighted in the following case. In *Re A (Children) Conjoined Twins: Surgical Separation* [2001] 2 WLR 480 Jodie and Mary were conjoined twins. Any separation would lead to saving Jodie's life (otherwise she would have died within six months) and the death of Mary (who would not have survived on her own). The parents objected to an operation, on religious grounds. This would have undoubtedly saved Jodie's life but led to the death of Mary. The Court of Appeal held that the operation should go ahead without the parents' consent.

Box 5.11 Case: Re R (A Minor) [1991] 4 All ER 177 CA

R, a 15-year-old girl, refused antipsychotic treatment for mental illness, which was intermittent, with violent and suicidal symptoms. She seemed lucid and rational at the time of refusal.

Held: The High Court held that R was incompetent and could receive compulsory treatment, though, nevertheless, only the court could override her refusal. Parents would have no right to make decisions on her behalf.

Section 47 of the National Assistance Act 1948 may be used in conjunction with the mental health compulsory admission powers to remove a person from their usual place of abode to a place of safety, which could be for treatment.

Research, consent and organ donation

Exceptions to the rule where patients may lack competence for consent include the following:

- unconscious patients,
- children below the age of majority – for exceptions see 'Fraser competence' in the *Gillick* case,
- confused patients – this may be due to condition of mental state,
- patients with mental health needs.

Box 5.12 Case: NHS Trust v DE [2013] EWHC 2562

A 41-year old man with learning disability, was deemed capable of consenting to sexual intercourse but could not make a proper decision on use of contraception. His girlfriend, who also had a learning disability and with whom he already had a child and the situation, was causing concern and anxiety for the couple. There was a concern that they would have another child if this was not controlled. The Court of Protection held, applying the issue of capacity under section 2 of the Mental Capacity Act 2005, that it was in the client's best interest to have a vasectomy.

Court of Protection, https://www.39essex.com/cop_cases/re-de/

When there is uncertainty due to the patient lacking capacity to consent, local guidelines (which are based on national guidelines) must be followed.

Box 5.13 Per Lord Goff in Airedale NHS Trust v. Bland [1993] AC 789

It is established that the principle of self-determination requires that respect be given to the wishes of the patient, so if an adult patient of sound mind refuses, however unreasonably, to consent to treatment or care by which his life would or might be prolonged, the doctors responsible for his care must give effect to his wishes, even though they do not consider it to be in his best interests to do so.

Research, consent and organ donation

The Nuremberg Code (1947) emerged as a result of the trial of that name, officially called *United States v Karl Brandt et al.* 'Known as the Doctors' Trial, [it] was prosecuted in 1946–47 against 23 doctors and administrators accused of organizing and participating in war crimes and crimes against humanity in the form of medical experiments and medical procedures inflicted on prisoners and civilians' (Harvard University, 2013). (confer on Chapter 2)

The crimes committed were experiments with people who were subjected to inhuman treatment by the Nazi high command. Examples of the experiments included in the indictments were:

1. High-altitude experiments, March–August 1942. Conducted for the German Air Force to investigate the effect of high-altitude flying; experiments were conducted at the Dachau Camp using a low-pressure chamber.

2. Freezing experiments, August 1942–May 1943. Conducted primarily for the German Air Force to investigate treatments for persons who had been severely chilled, using prisoners at the Dachau Camp.
3. Malaria experiments, February 1942–April 1945. Conducted to test immunization for and treatment of malaria; experiments were conducted on more than 1,000 prisoners at Dachau.

Subsequently, an international agreement was put in place to regulate medical experiments and clinical trials. The Code has ten requirements, among them:

> 1. The voluntary consent of the human subject is absolutely essential. This means that the person involved should have legal capacity to give consent: should be so situated as to be able to exercise free power of choice without the intervention of any element of force, fraud, deceit, duress, overreaching, or other ulterior form of constraint or coercion and should have sufficient knowledge and comprehension of the elements of the subject matter involved as to enable him to make an understanding and enlightened decision.
> (Trials of War Criminals before the Nuremberg Military Tribunals, 1946–49)

Research may involve clinical trials, which not only require consent but may also be regulated by contract law, where a participant is paid money in exchange for participation. Depending on the terms of agreement, the courts may not view favourably where there is an underlying contractual agreement. In the event of adverse reaction, the defendant is entitled to a defence of *volenti non fit injuria*, translated from Latin as 'to a willing person, no injury is done'. This means that potentially, any damages awarded for personal injury may be reduced substantially as a result. Where, however, a contractual exclusion of liability clause is included, the defendant cannot use the above principle or an exclusion or limitation of liability clause where a person is injured seriously or killed as a result of the defendant's negligent actions (Unfair Contract Terms Act 1977). Others, however, see consent in research as a way for the researcher to transfer some of the risk to the informed subject (Alderson and Goodey, 1998).

A sufficient degree of information is vital to enable the participants to make an informed choice. In the following case, had participants known the adverse and dangerous effects and impact of the experiments, they would not have agreed. One leading example is the Tuskegee syphilis study, where clinical research in Alabama between 1932 and 1972 involved a large group of black males, about 600 in total. Of this group, 400 were deliberately infected with syphilis (the rest was a control group of 200 which was uninfected). The aim was to find out 'whether blacks reacted to syphilis in the same way as whites, and to determine how long a human being can live with untreated syphilis. The men that were used in the research, most of them uneducated sharecroppers were left untreated with syphilis and suffered tremendously in the hands of doctors from the US Public Health Service' (Ogungbure, 2011, p. 75).

Sections 30–35 of the Mental Capacity Act 2005 now provide for advocacy in research, with additional safeguards (Section 33) for protection of any person lacking in consent who may be involved in research:

> 2) Nothing may be done to, or in relation to, him in the course of the research
>   (a) to which he appears to object (whether by showing signs of resistance or otherwise) except where what is being done is intended to protect him from harm or to reduce or prevent pain or discomfort, or

(b) which would be contrary to
   (i)   an advance decision of his which has effect, or
   (ii) any other form of statement made by him and not subsequently with-
         drawn, of which R is aware.

(Section 33(2) of Mental Capacity Act 2005)

Organs may be donated for research purposes or to save lives; either way, consent should be obtained before this. Following the Liverpool and Bristol inquiry reports, the Health Service Circular HSC 2001/023 (Department of Health, 2001d, p. 4) suggests that

> Review of the law on the taking and use of human organs and tissue is currently in progress as part of the follow-up to the Liverpool and Bristol inquiry reports. Pending the outcome of this review, the model consent for treatment forms do not yet include a section on consent for the use of tissue removed during medical procedures, but the model policy makes clear that NHS organisations must have clear procedures in place to ensure that patients have the opportunity to refuse permission for such use if they wish.

As nurses are becoming more involved in research, they need to ensure that consent is properly obtained, especially if they are assisting others who may not have properly obtained this (RCN, 2005). Research involving human organs must always be in writing:

5) Consent in writing for the purposes of subsection (3) is only valid if –
   (a) it is signed by the person concerned in the presence of at least one witness who attests the signature,
   (b) it is signed at the direction of the person concerned, in his presence and in the presence of at least one witness who attests the signature, or
   (c) it is contained in a will of the person concerned made in accordance with the requirements of –
        (i) section 9 of the Wills Act 1837 (c. 26)

(Human Tissue Act 2004)

One important change introduced by the above statute in this area of law is that any such properly constituted consent may not be overruled by family members. Another important area is highlighted in the scandals involving illegal organ storage and use for research. The Human Tissue Act (HTA) 2004 took effect on 1 September 2006, outlawing the following practices:

- the removal or storage of human tissue without prior consent, following the Alder Hey scandal.
- the taking and testing of DNA without consent;
- trafficking of organs.

The above offences now attract penalties ranging from a fine to three years' imprisonment or both. The NHS Plan (Department of Health, 2000) also gives further guidance on good practice and the need to obtain consent in research. The NHS Constitution (2015) aims to promote patient-centred care and putting the patient at the centre of decision-making.

Box 5.14 Thinking point

A 21-year-old man (with an organ donor card) who has been in a persistent vegetative state (PVS) since suffering brain damage following a road traffic accident has been on a ventilator, and a decision has been made to switch off the ventilator. The family has been approached but is strongly opposed to organ donation.

Consider the legal and ethical implications of organ donation in light of the proposed changes to the law on presumed consent, and in this case (on presumed consent).

Human Transportation (Wales) Act 2013

The aim of the Act is to increase the number of organs and tissues available for transplant. This will benefit the people of Wales by reducing the number of people dying whilst waiting for a suitable organ to become available and improving the lives of others.

(Wales Government 2013)

In respect of consent in organ donation, it is difficult when the decision is not a simple matter of self-determination but a decision which may impact on the views of family members and their rights to object. These objections may be based on cultural or religious grounds. The National Patient Safety Agency (2011) now regulates the NHS research framework through the Health Research Authority.

Conclusion

In practice, it is difficult for clinicians to determine whether a patient giving consent does so of their own accord on the basis of reasoned judgement or due to influence from others, such as close family members, friends or other clinicians. What is important is that unless it is an emergency, the patient should whenever possible be given a sufficient degree of information to enable them to make a choice on whether to accept treatment or not – the opportunity to deliberate and make an important decision to consent to treatment or, likewise, decline it. They should never feel under pressure from nurses, family members or other healthcare professionals. Difficulties may arise when patients do not wish to have this information because of ignorance, fear of coming to terms with any outcome, perhaps in denial, or they may not wish to know (as far as risks of an operation are concerned), or they may believe that the nurse or doctor knows 'what is best for them'. The role of the nurse should be to ensure that where possible, the patient's right to informed consent is safeguarded, unless they lack mental capacity – establishing this is always going to be a challenge for the nurse. No decisions should be made about the patient's treatment without their involvement. With regard to treatment, the ethics of self-determination and autonomy have long been recognized in common law.

References

Adults with Incapacity (Scotland) Act (2008).
Airedale NHS Trust v Bland [1993] AC 789.
Alderson P and Goodey C. Theories of consent. *BMJ* 1998; 317: 1313–15.

Beatty v Cullingworth Q.B. Unreported [1896] 44 CENT. L.J. 153 (s896).

Beauchamp TL and Childress JF. *Principles of biomedical ethics*, 7th ed. New York: Oxford University Press, 2013.

Blackburn S. *Being good: A short introduction to ethics*. Oxford: Oxford University Press, 2001.

Campbell A, Gillett G and Jones G. *Medical ethics*. Oxford: Oxford University Press, 2001.

Chester v Afshar [2004] UKHL 41.

Children Act 1989, Section 1.

Control of Diseases Act 1984.

Department of Health (2000) Post-mortem examination. Advice from the Chief Medical Officer. Available online at: www.doh.gov.uk/orgretentionadvic (accessed on 20th April 2011).

Department of Health (2001a) *Guidance for clinicians: Model policy for consent to examination or treatment*. Available online at: www.dh.gov.uk/PolicyAndGuidance/HealthAndSocial-CareTopics/Consent/ConsentGeneralInformation/fs/en (accessed on 21st August 2006).

Department of Health (2001b) *Good practice in consent implementation guide*. Crown.

Department of Health (22nd November 2001d) *Health service circular*. HSC 2001/023, p. 4.

Doyal L. Good clinical practice and informed consent are inseparable. *Heart* 2002; 87: 103–5. Available online at: www.heart.bmj.com/cgi/content/abstract/87/2/103 (accessed on 22nd October 2019).

Fletcher L and Buka. *A legal framework for caring*. Basingstoke: Palgrave Macmillan, 1999.

Furrow D. *Ethics: Key concepts in philosophy*. London: Continuum, 2005.

F v West Berkshire Health Authority and Another (Mental Health Act Commission Intervening) [1989] 2 All ER at 545.

General Medical Council (2008) Consent guidance: Patients and doctors making decisions together. Available online at: https://www.gmc-uk.org//media/documents/Consent___English_0617.pdf_48903482.pdf (accessed on 3rd October 2019).

General Medical Council. *Seeking patients' consent: The ethical considerations*. London: GMC, 1999.

Giliker P and Bethwith S. *Tort*, 2nd ed. London: Sweet and Maxwell, 2011.

Gillick v West Norfolk and Wisbech Area Health Authority [1985] 3 All ER 492.

Hart HLA. *Punishment and responsibility*. Oxford: Oxford University Press, 1968.

Harvard University. Indictment in trials of war criminals, 16–18. Available online at: http://nuremberg.law.harvard.edu/nurTranscript/TranscriptSearches/tran_about.php (accessed on 10th July 2019).

Health and Social Care Act 2008.

Hoffman D and Rowe J. *Human rights in the UK: An introduction to the Human Rights Act 1998*, 4th ed. London: Pearson Longman, 2013.

Human Rights Act 1998, Articles 3, 5(e) 8.

Human Transportation (Wales) Act 2013.

Human Tissue Act 2004.

Legal Capacity (Scotland) Act 1991. Sections 2 (4).

Mental Capacity Act 2005, sections 2, 4(2), 20, 30–35.

Mental Capacity Act 2005 (Adults with Incapacity (Scotland) Act 2000).

Mental Health Act 1983. Available online at: www.doh.gov.uk/mentalhealth/ (accessed 6 July 2019).

Mental Health Act 1983, Sections, 56–64. 93, 93(1) (b) 94(2), 95, -98.

Mental Health Act 2007.

Mental Health (Care and Treatment) (Scotland) Act 2003.

Mill JS. *On liberty*, Everyman edition. London: JM Dent, 1993. National Patient Safety Agency (Amendment no. 3). Directions 2011 published on 1 December 2011. Available online at: http://webarchive.nationalarchives.gov.uk/20111202162649/http://dh.gov.uk/health/2011/12/creation-hra (accessed on 12 September 2019).

Montgomery v Lanarkshire Health Board [2015] UKSC 11.

National Assistance Act 1948, Section 47.

NHS Constitution (2015) Available online at: https://www.gov.uk/government/publications/the-nhs-constitution-for-england (accessed on 4th August 2019).

NHS Trust v DE [2013] EWHC 2562.

Nozick R. *Anarchy, state, and utopia.* New York: Basic Books, 1974.

Nursing and Midwifery Council (2018) Professional standards of practice and behaviour for nurses, midwives and nursing associates. Available online at: https://www.nmc.org.uk/standards/code/ (accessed on 5th October 2019).

O'Brien v Cunard SS Co. [1891] 28 NE 266.

Offences against the Person Act 1861.

Ogungbure AA. The Tuskegee syphilis study: Some ethical reflections, thought and practice. *Journal of the Philosophical Association of Kenya (PAK)* 2011; 3(2): 75–92.

Re A (Children) Conjoined Twins: Surgical Separation [2001] 2 WLR 480.

Re C Test/Re C Advice: Refusal of Treatment [1994] 1 WLR 290.

Re R (A Minor) [1991] 4 All ER 177 CA.

Re S [1994] 2 FLR 1065.

Re T [1992] 9 BMLR 46.

Royal College of Nursing Research Society. *Informed consent in health and social care research.* RCN Guidance for Nurses. 2005.

Schloendorff v Society of New York Hospital 211 NY; 105 NE 92, 93 [1914]; 106 NE 93; NY [1914].

Sidaway v Board of Governors of the Bethlem Royal Hospital and the Maudsley Hospital [1985] AC 871.

St George's Healthcare National Health Service Trust v S (no. 2) reported in The Times Law Report of 3 August 1998.

Thompson I, Melia K and Boyd K. *Nursing ethics*, 6th ed. London: Churchill Livingstone, 2006.

Trials of War Criminals before the Nuremberg Military Tribunals under Control Council Law no. 10. Nuremberg, October 1946–April 1949. Washington: U.S. Government Printing Office (n.d.), vol. 2, pp. 181–2. Available online at: www.cirp.org/library/ethics/nuremberg/.

Unfair Contract Terms Act 1977.

Wales Government (2013) Available online at: http://wales.gov.uk/topics/health/nhswales/majorhealth/organ/?lang=en

WHO. *Ethics of the health systems: Report of the third futures forum for high-level decision-makers.* Stockholm, Sweden, 27–28 June 2002.

WHO (2003) Available online at: https://apps.who.int/iris/handle/10665/107449 (accessed on 14 September 2019).

Williamson v East London and City Health Authority, HA [1998], Lloyds Reports, Med 6, [1990].

Wills Act 1837 (c. 26).

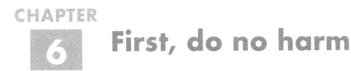

First, do no harm

Chapter outline

Introduction
Background to safety
Health and safety at work
Manual handling and product liability
Universal precautions and infection control
Vicarious liability and clinical negligence
Occupier's liability
Safe medicines management and administration
Conclusion

Introduction

This chapter applies bioethical principles and legal frameworks which are related to safety and impacting the quality of care. It should be the priority of all healthcare providers to ensure that they comply with Health and Safety legislation and that service users are kept safe. Human factors define quality within a clinical environment and the employer-employee relationship may affect the quality of care. Patients' rights are at the centre of health and safety, and are affected by the expected conduct of healthcare professionals and others who deliver care. Although it is not always obvious, the professional caring relationship also as contractual implication under employment law. This is between the healthcare provider (employer) and the nurse, healthcare assistants or other health and social care professionals. Nurses should be guided by the Nursing and Midwifery Council (NMC) standards of care as well as the requirement to comply with health safety legislation.

Background to safety

Bioethical principles apply directly to aspects of safety, and breach of them may have legal consequences.

- *Beneficence* and *non-maleficence*: Both these are applicable in order to ensure that the patient benefits and is not harmed by the nurse's negligent actions or omissions.

- *Fairness:* Avoid discrimination and ensure a fair distribution of scarce resources. This means that a patient's safety must not be compromised by preferential treatment of others.
- *Autonomy:* Failure to properly obtain consent or to facilitate the patient's decision-making may mean that a patient is harmed through violation of this human right.

It may be a useful starting point to consider the following maxim and observation as a point of focus:

> The very first requirement in a hospital is that it should do the sick no harm.
> (Florence Nightingale 1820–1910)

The Francis Report (2013) identified some organizational cultural problems within the NHS and made several key recommendations included with *five key points*:

1. "Common culture" has been proposed throughout the NHS
2. The report places emphasis on the creation of a "safety culture"
3. An organisation should have shared values from top management to frontline staff
4. The NHS must have strong, consistent leadership to motivate staff
5. Everyone employed by the NHS should have a "questioning attitude, a rigorous approach and good communication skills"

(Francis, 2013)

    With major inquiries come publicity, and it is clear that the expectations of the public have been on the rise since the Patients' Charter (1992). Demographic changes show that with improved medicine and quality of life, people are living longer. It is, however, also clear that there have also been several failures when patients were harmed. One example was the Royal Bristol Inquiry (2001).

    The NHS Constitution (2015) aims to empower the patient and improve the quality of care, so the service user is at the heart of the care provision. From the patient's perspective, over the years, there has been a rise in litigations. The Francis Report (2013) aimed to promote the duty of candour in order for NHS staff to learn from incidents. If a patient who is at risk is harmed, it is incumbent for managers to carry out a route-cause analysis to find out what went wrong and who was responsible for any human factors which resulted in the safety breach which caused the harm and what lessons have been learnt,

    The NHS has defined quality as set out by Lord Darzi in 2008. This requires the following criteria should be met::

- patient safety (doing no harm to patients)
- patient experience (care should be characterised by compassion, dignity and respect);
- effectiveness of care (to be measured using survival rates, complication rates, measures of clinical improvement, and patient-reported outcome measures.

(Kingsfund, 2008)

Patient safety is one of the three strands of the NHS Quality Agenda, and nurses have a vital role to play in the promotion and maintenance of safe clinical environments. The NPSA defined levels of risk based on consequence scoring as

1. Negligible
2. Minor
3. Moderate
4. Major
5. Catastrophic

(NPSA, 2008)

There are different levels of accountability in law which may be applicable in consideration of safety.

Professional accountability – NMC Code (2018)

The four themes are all relevant.

- prioritize people, which means that care-delivery should always place the patient at the centre of everything they do (NHS Constitution, 2015);
- practise effectively, relates to accountability and means that healthcare professionals should be able to justify their actions;
- preserve safety is the key one and requires risk assessment and risk management to ensure safe practice in order to ensure that patients are not harmed; and
- promote professionalism and trust, defines the nurse's role as a professional, and this relates to the above three themes.

Human Rights Act 1998

Civil law – duty of care to ensure that no person is injured as a result of our negligent actions, may sue for damages
Criminal law – prosecution for battery/health by police
Employment law – breach of terms of contract – employees
Health & Safety at Work Act 1974 – harm in the workplace, this will be explored in the next section below.

It is possible, in an informal caring relationship where family and friends are involved either exclusively or in partnership with 'employed' health and social care workers. In both types of settings, the users' safety should never be compromised, and everything should be done to promote professionals working in collaboration with informal carers to ensure patient safety. Factors which may affect the patient's 'best interests' will be considered in the context of duty of care in ethics as well as health and safety and employment law.

As well as ethical considerations above, a nurse owes the patient a duty of care in common law. There is an obligation to ensure that the patient is not harmed by their negligent actions or omissions. This principle underpins liability for harm in the law of torts or delict (in Scotland), notwithstanding professional regulations by bodies such as the Nursing and Midwifery Council (NMC), General Medical Council (for medical staff) or Health and Care Professions Council (for other health and social care professionals). Based on the assumption that an employee undertakes a role voluntarily, it stands to reason that on appointment, they will be expected to meet the minimum requirements of the role in question as well as the terms. Likewise, the employer also honours the contractual terms and the conditions of service (Selwyn, 2011).

In search of a definition of nursing, the International Council for nurses could not have suggested a more fittingone, and there is an expectation that:

> nursing encompasses autonomous and collaborative care of individuals of all ages, families, groups and communities, sick or well and in all settings. Nursing includes the promotion of health, prevention of illness, and the care of ill, disabled and dying people. Advocacy, promotion of a safe environment, research, participation in shaping health policy and in patient and health systems management, and education are also key nursing roles.
>
> (International Council of Nurses)

Health and safety at work

Health and safety is a broad employment law concept with statutory criminal liability, with its main objective as safeguarding patients, as well as staff and visitors. A victim does not need to prove negligence on the part of the owner of a building. For example, health and safety also requires the employer to manage substances hazardous to health, subject to the Control of Substances Hazardous to Health Regulations (COSHH) 1999. The Ministry of Defence may be exempt under Section 17 of the above statutory instrument. This means that employers are required to reasonably control and protect patients, staff and visitors from exposure to hazardous substances to prevent ill health.

As many as

- *1.4 million* working people suffering from a work-related illness
- *2,526* mesothelioma deaths due to past asbestos exposures (2017)
- *147* workers killed at work
- *581,000* working people sustaining an injury at work according to the Labour Force Survey
- *69,208* injuries to employees reported under RIDDOR

(HSE (2018/19))

It is, however, not clear how many patients died as a direct result of health and safety-related accidents. A hospital looking after patients has the duty to ensure the safe storage of hazardous substances as these may injure a person who comes into contact with them, particularly in a case of a confused patient or children. It is observed, nevertheless, that the chance of a victim winning a case under health and safety legislation are better than under the normal rules of civil claim in tort (Mandelstam, 2017). The reality is that (as discussed above) damages are much lower.

The Health and Safety at Work Act (HASAWA) 1974 is the key statute in managing risk in the health and safety area. A hazard is the potential to cause harm, while risk is the likelihood of harm to take place depending on certain circumstances. The Safety Representatives and Safety Committees Regulations 1977 and the Health and Safety (Consultation with Employees) Regulations 1996 require employers to, inform, and consult with, employees in good time on matters relating to their health and safety. Employee representatives, either appointed by recognised trade unions under (a) or elected under (b) may make representations to their employer on matters affecting the health and safety of those they represent.

(HSE, http://www.hse.gov.uk/violence/law.htm)

This area is regulated by the Health and Safety Executive (HSE) through its HSE Commission, which is responsible for health and safety regulation in the United Kingdom. Together with local authorities (environmental health) the HSE is the enforcing authority and supports the commission. The employer's specific responsibilities in this area include maintaining a safe system of work as well as risk management including a duty to provide appropriate equipment and to ensure appropriate staff training.

Box 6.1 HSE case study 1: Hospital trust improves floor cleaning after a slip

A hospital worker opened the door of a meeting room and stepped into the corridor. She slipped and fell, as the vinyl floor had just been cleaned and was still wet. Although she was not seriously injured, this was largely a matter of chance – there was the potential for a serious injury on another occasion.

An HSE inspector happened to witness the incident and immediately made enquiries about how floor cleaning operations were managed by the trust. He was sufficiently concerned to issue an improvement notice. The main concerns were:

- wet mopping on vinyl floor – likely to be slippery if left wet,
- no suitable barriers to prevent people stepping onto the wet floor (single cone was in use – insufficient given large area being cleaned),
- direct access from adjoining rooms onto wet area – no warning for people exiting the rooms,
- floor cleaning carried out at unsuitable time (dinner time on main access route to canteen),
- new cleaner – not adequately trained or supervised.

The improvement notice required the setting up of suitable cleaning regimes and safe systems of work to prevent pedestrians stepping onto a wet floor. It also required the trust to set up a system to ensure that the new procedures were working, including appointing someone to be responsible for monitoring them.

The trust responded promptly and positively to comply with the notice. They put in place improved systems and procedures, including the following:

- retraining of staff on use of conventional mopping systems,
- cleaning floors in small sections, followed by dry mopping,
- effective use of cones and barriers,
- better demonstration of the training methods and systems of work used by contract cleaners,
- trust-wide circulation of the lessons learnt from this incident and the remedial actions taken.

HSE (2013) http://www.hse.gov.uk/slips/experience/floorcleaning.htm by kind permission of the Health and safety executive.

The employer is duty-bound under health and safety legislation to identify hazards and risks, through risk management and preventative actions (Ridley, 2008), as well as (evaluative) risk assessment. This is covered by Section 2(1) of the HASAWA 1974. (See above.)

Box 6.2 Thinking point

A patient is admitted from a residential home to a surgical urology ward. He is an 89-year-old male resident who has a history of dementia, and he gets more confused at night-time and attempts to get out of bed several times, demanding to 'go home to see his mother'. At night-time, staff were concerned about the possibility of him climbing out of bed and falling since there is only three of them: two qualified nurses and a healthcare assistant. His daughter, who was the next of kin, suggested that nurses use cot sides as a precaution as her father was not very steady on his feet and had already had several falls in the home prior to admission.

Consider application of the Liberty Protection Safeguards (2019) (formerly DoLS)

However, in respect of the nurse as an employee, Section 7 of the HASAWA 1974 requires them to take reasonable measures to ensure their own safety and that of others, primarily the patient, other staff, as well as visitors, in order to ensure that their work environment is safe. They must also avoid risk to health in respect of the patient, themselves, colleagues and visitors. In addition to the requirements of health and safety laws, they must avoid risk by adhering to local safety policy and instructions of their employer as well as report any unsafe practice. In addition, it is impossible to forestall every eventuality in aiming to eliminate potential hazards. There is nevertheless a requirement for a proper risk assessment with the following requirements.

For example, use of bed rails is an important aspect of safety which needs systematic and thorough risk assessment. Nurses should ensure the following (HSE, 2013):

- They (bed rails) are only provided when they are the right solution to prevent falls.
- A risk assessment is carried out by a competent person considering the bed occupant, the bed, mattresses, bed rails and all associated equipment.
- The rail is suitable for the bed and mattress.
- The mattress fits snugly between the rails.
- The rail is correctly fitted, secure, regularly inspected and maintained.
- Gaps that could cause entrapment of neck, head and chest are eliminated.
- Staff are trained in the risks and safe use of bed rails.

The courts apply the 'reasonableness' test in determining the best use of available resources in order to minimize rather than eliminate hazards (*Donoghue v Stevenson* [1932] UKHL 100). In defence, a healthcare provider, as occupier of premises, will need to demonstrate that they followed a set procedure and did everything reasonable in order to minimize harm through a risk assessment. In the event of a patient suffering harm as a result of negligence, however, exclusion of liability clauses may not limit liability in negligence if there is resulting injury or death, under Section 16 of the Unfair Contract Terms Act 1977. In all other cases strict liability applies.

There is now a legal requirement to report work-related accidents under the HSE Reporting of Injuries, Disease and Dangerous Occurrences (RIDDOR) 2013 first passed as the Reporting of Injuries, Disease and Dangerous Occurrences Regulations 1995. The classification of accidents requiring to be reported falls within the following categories (Croner CCH Group, 2002, pp. 21–22):

- death,
- major injuries to employees such as a fall, resulting in sickness of at least three days,
- other significant injury of non-employees requiring hospital treatment,
- specified diseases,
- specified dangerous occurrences including escape of noxious substances.

An estimated 591,000 workers had an accident at work in 2011–12, and 212,000 of these injuries led to over three days' absence from work and 156,000 to over seven days' (LFS) (HSE, 2013).

The employer should also manage substances hazardous to health subject to the Control of Substances Hazardous to Health Regulations (COSHH) 1999. The Ministry of Defence may be exempt under Section 17 of the above statutory instrument. This means that employers are required to reasonably control and protect patients, staff and visitors from exposure to hazardous substances to prevent ill health.

A care provider has a duty to ensure the safe storage of hazardous substances as these may injure a person who comes into contact with them, particularly in a case of a confused patient or children. It is observed nevertheless that the chance of a victim winning a case under health and safety legislation are better than under the normal rules of civil claim in tort (Mandelstam, 2017). The reality is that (as discussed above) damages are much lower.

Manual handling and product liability

This is another important aspect of health and safety legislation safeguarding the patient's welfare for those with mobility needs. Nurses play an important part in this process. As well as the common law duty of care based on the Health and Safety at Work Act 1974, there is a supplementary regulation on the manual handling in the form of Manual Handling Operations Regulations (MHOR) 1992. The aim during any risk assessment should be 'weighing up the risk of injury against the cost or effort required to introduce new measures. Doing nothing can only be justified if the cost of measures greatly outweighs the risk' (Royal College of Nursing (RCN), 2002, p. 4). Supplementary safety legislation must operate within the framework of the HASAWA 1974 (Mandelstam, 2017). The Manual Handling Operations Regulations: Lifting Operations and Lifting Equipment Regulations 1998 Health and Safety Commission (HSC) includes regulation of the inspection and use of appropriateness of equipment used for moving and handling patients.

EC Directive 85/374/EEC was intended to apply to all member states in its entirety, in response to the needs of a victim facing the uphill struggle in establishing negligence and product liability. Prior to this Consumer Protection Act 1987 (Product Liability) (Modification) Order 2000 and the Consumer Protection Act 1987 (Product Liability) (Modification) (Scotland) Order 2001, a plaintiff must prove that a manufacturer was negligent before they can claim for damages, now subject to Part I of this statute, on product liability. Injury caused by defective products removes the need to prove negligence, also providing strict liability. The causes for litigation include all defective biomedical equipment and medication which are covered by the Consumer Protection Act 1987. This may be used against a drug manufacturer when a patient has suffered resulting harm.

Universal precautions and infection control

The principle of duty of care to patients is applicable to cases of infection control and safety, as hospitals are required to minimize the risk by taking reasonable measures to prevent harm where possible. There is a reasonable expectation that nurses will follow established procedures in infection control. negligence arises from a breach of duty of care if the nurse's conduct falls below expected standards, with resulting harm to patients. The employer and/or the nurse may be held liable, although in practice the employer is likely to be sued on the basis of vicarious liability, discussed below. Hospital-acquired infections (HAI) are on the rise:

> The overall prevalence of healthcare-associated infections in all acute care hospitals surveyed in the Health Protection Agency's National Point Prevalence Survey was 6.4% in 2011 compared to 8.2% in 2006.
>
> (NICE, 2015)

Box 6.3 Thinking point

John, a newly qualified staff nurse on an acute medicine for care of the elderly ward, is concerned about the ward which has a poor reputation and a high level of complaints with the following problems:

1   There is a chronic staff shortage on the ward, and the ward sister says she has raised this with senior nurse managers, who have done little about it.
2   Recently, he witnessed the sister and another nurse using a method which was not recommended for moving a patient, but he is not sure what to do for fear of reprisals.
3   There are four cases of methicillin-resistant *Staphylococcus aureus* (MRSA) on the ward, and he thinks this may be linked to a generally very poor standard of hygiene on the ward.
    (a) Consider your employer's guidelines on infection control.
    (b) Consider national guidelines.

It is clear that in order to contain some infections, patients may need to be nursed in isolation for the purpose of managing and minimizing cross-infection. On the other hand, there may also be a need to balance overall interests of all patients against those of the isolated patients. There are ethical issues here, as patients may complain on a limitation of their freedom by being isolated with a possible infringement of their human rights under Articles 4 (related to their freedom) and 14 (in respect of their right not to be discriminated against) of the Human Rights Act 1998, if they feel that they have been provided a lower standard of care. The nurse is required to show that they have provided a reasonable standard of care expected of their peers, following the Bolam Test.

Box 6.4 Case: Bolam v Friern Hospital Management Committee [1957] 1 WLR 582

The claimant underwent electro-convulsive therapy (ECT) treatment for endogenous depression. The anaesthetist did not administer any relaxant drugs and the claimant suffered convulsions and fractures. There were divided opinions amongst professionals regarding the effectiveness and risk of the practice of giving a muscle relaxant drug. One view suggested a very small risk of death, and another school of thought recognized a small risk of fractures, which is what happened with the claimant. The claimant argued a breach of duty by the doctor in not administering the muscle relaxant drug.

Held: It was held by the House of Lords that the doctor was not in breach of duty. 'A medical professional is not guilty of negligence if he (or she) has acted in accordance with a practice accepted as proper by a responsible body of medical men skilled in that particular art .... Putting it the other way around, a man (or woman) is not negligent, if he (or she) is acting in accordance with such a practice, merely because there is a body of opinion who would take a contrary view'. From a health and safety perspective, the hospital as employer has a duty of care to staff and as occupier to patients to ensure that there are adequate resources and staffing levels when delivering care. There has been a suggestion of a correlation between poor nursing staffing levels and mortality levels (Needleman and Buerhaus, 2003) and as a part of unsafe practice (Aiken et al., 2002). The nurse should engage in safe practice on the grounds that they owe a duty of care to the patient, and therefore a breach of that duty may give rise to damages in tort for the harmed patient.

Since 2002, annual figures showed that 70,000 people were estimated to die from infection-related deaths (DoH, 2002), with similar trends as shown by more recent figures, with a total of 2,500,331 of deaths related to MRSA and *Staphylococcus aureus* between 2003 and 2011 (ONS, 2013). It is important for trusts to restore patient confidence by ensuring the cleanliness of ward areas as a way of controlling and minimizing infections. Two comparative surveys between 2002 and 2004 showed that patient ratings on cleanliness had fallen by 3 per cent, from 51 to 48 per cent, for 'very clean' and by 2 per cent, from 41 to 39 per cent, for 'fairly clean', respectively (UNISON, 2004). All organizations should ensure they are complying with legislation that is relevant to managing the risks to employees from exposure to blood-borne viruses. Particular attention should be paid to (HSE, 2013):

- providing written policies and procedures with clear lines of accountability;
- carrying out suitable and sufficient risk assessments, following the COSHH hierarchy, including use of safer devices;
- assessing the contribution and role of competent advisors, that is, health and safety, risk management, occupational health and infection control;
- ensuring staff are informed of the risks and implementing control measures, including reporting sharps injuries;
- ensuring suitable monitoring and auditing arrangements are in place.

The cost of infectious diseases is significant to health care in the UK, accounting for 7 per cent of deaths, with annual costs of £30 billion (Houses of Parliament Parliamentary Office, 2017).

Vicarious liability and clinical negligence

There is a presumption in law that an employer takes credit for the positive actions of their employees; accordingly, it stands to reason therefore that they (employer) should also bear any loss resulting from negligent actions of their employees, based on the principle of 'vicarious liability'. Given that this is the case in a caring environment, the employer should therefore take responsibility for the negative aspects as well. This includes the actions of commission or omissions carried out by employees (in the course of their employment). It stands to reason therefore that the employer should bear the leading and ultimate responsibility for not only safeguarding patients' rights but also owing anyone who comes on their premises, such as patients, staff and family members, a duty of care by providing a safe working environment under Section 2 of the Health and Safety at Work Act 1974, as well as ensuring the welfare of the patients. Employees are nevertheless expected to follow reasonable orders and also have a duty of care under Section 7 of the Health and Safety at Work Act 1974.

Box 6.5 Thinking point

Jane had been working as a district nurse and team leader in the community for the preceding ten years managing a caseload of mostly elderly patients with long-term conditions. This included Mr Smith (aged 90 years) and his wife (86 years old). He was a retired engineer who had a diagnosis of diabetes Type 1 (on insulin) and Parkinson's disease, and had been recently transferred to Jane's caseload following a colleague's retirement about four weeks prior to this. There had been no proper handover as the nurse who had been looking after this patient had gone off sick before retiring on health grounds. Jane assigned one of her nurses, Jill, for direct care. During the first assessment Jill was advised by the patient that he was self-caring apart from weekly home help, mainly cleaning the house and shopping, as well as meals on wheels. The couple managed with mutual support with occasional help from family members.

The district nurse came in every day to give him his insulin injection. One morning the patient was seen by another new staff nurse, Maria. She had many years nursing experience in her country of origin but only eight months' post-adaptation experience in the UK. She speaks English with slight difficulty in understanding, though she usually works well, with minimum supervision. On the day in question a year one nursing student had been temporarily allocated to Maria as the student's mentor was on half-term leave. Under her supervision, the student nurse was instructed to draw up 8 ml (millilitres) of long-acting insulin, instead of 8 IU (international units), and she promptly administered the injection. (She used the wrong syringe as the patient had run out of his own stock.) Soon after they left, the patient went into a hypoglycaemic attack. His wife called for an ambulance, which arrived within 30 minutes of the call. Attempts to resuscitate him were unsuccessful. At the inquest, the student nurse said she remembered the patient saying he had a supply of his own syringes and that this was the wrong syringe. she did mention the difference in needles to Maria, who told her that she knew what she was doing.

1   What risk assessments should have been carried out prior to this?
2   Consider your employer's policy on management and administration of medicines.

Based on the legal doctrine, *'respondeat superior'* on vicarious liability, the law presumes that an employer is liable for any actions or omissions which are incurred by the employee 'in the course of their employment'. In a few cases which have gone to law did decisions go against this general principle, when it comes to employee acting 'outside the course of their employment'. It is the employer's legal responsibility to issue terms and conditions of service to the employee, within two months of employment, as regulated by the Employment Rights Act (ERA) 1996, which was amended by the Employment Relations Act (ERA) 1999 and the Employment Act 2002. If a workforce has good working conditions and nurses are working in a safe environment, they are more likely to deliver safe care for patients.

The terms of employment are usually in writing, though this is not necessary as custom and practice may be sufficient to establish a contract of employment, in the event of a dispute going to an employment tribunal. This means that where terms of a contract of employment are not written, the court may exercise its prerogative in interpreting implied terms as evidenced by the actions and relationship between an employer and employee (Phillips and Scott, 2008). It may, however, be more difficult to establish an unwritten contract if this is not written.

There are two of types of employment contracts, that is, a contract of services and a contract for services:

1. A *contract of services* is the most common type of agreement for most nurses in employment, whether as full-time or part-time. An employee works to an agreed contract or agreement with specific terms for a specified wage or salary, and this is easier to determine liability. In cases where, however, an employee acts illegally or outside the scope of their work (or practice), the question arises whether the employer should be vicariously liable. The point in issue is illustrated by the following case:

Box 6.6 Case: Lister and Others v Hall [2001] UKHL 22

A warden who was an employee at a boarding school to look after young boys instead abused them.

Held: Although the defendant carried out criminal acts which were not authorized by his employer, this was nevertheless 'in the course of his employment' and therefore the employer was liable under the principle of vicarious liability.

---

2. A *contract for services*, on the other hand, applies to agency or hired workers who are either self-employed through an agency or working for themselves. To illustrate the problems faced by agency staff (who are self-employed), there may be difficulties in establishing liability. This means that in contract law, a principal for an agency nurse may be sued for the actions of their agency worker, though this is difficult in practice unless it can be proved that they knowingly colluded with the agency nurse or acted negligently. An example of this principle is illustrated in the following case:

Box 6.7 Case: Weddall v Barchester Healthcare Ltd [2012] EWCA Civ 25

Mr Weddall was a deputy manager at a care home. One evening while on duty, Mr Weddall telephoned Mr Marsh, a senior health assistant, who was off duty and asked him if he was willing to work a nightshift as another employee had turned in sick.

Mr Marsh was drunk and became angry and upset on the call, as he thought Mr Weddall was mocking him. Twenty minutes later Mr Marsh cycled to the care home and (hopping mad) violently attacked Mr Weddall. Mr Marsh was sentenced to 15 months imprisonment for a criminal assault. Mr Weddall brought a claim against Barchester Homes, alleging that it was vicariously liable for Mr Marsh's actions.

A county court judge held that Mr Marsh had acted personally (i.e. he was not carrying out his employment duties at the time but rather acting for his own reasons) and it would not be fair and just to hold Barchester Homes vicariously liable. Mr Weddall appealed to the Court of Appeal.

The Appeal Court found that Mr Marsh's actions were 'an independent venture ... separate and distinct from Marsh's employment as a Senior Health Assistant at a care home'.

http://www.hempsons.co.uk/news/violence-and-vicarious-liability-2

There is a presumption in law that an employer is in a more financially privileged position in comparison to an employee. This therefore makes the employer the primary target for litigation in seeking substantial compensation for harm in tort or delict (Scots law) for a victim of clinical negligence. It is nevertheless possible for the employee to be jointly cited as co-defendant in a civil action for damages for clinical negligence.

The employer is nevertheless within their right to indemnify their own loss by suing a negligent employee in turn as they seek to make good any losses resulting from the employee's negligent actions (in the event of an employee acting negligently by failing to follow existing policy and procedure). In most cases, nurses may also be indemnified through their union insurance. However, if it can be established that in the course of employment an employee was following established (employer) procedures with resulting injury to a patient, then clearly the responsibility for negligence will lie with the employer. This principle was applied as 'an implied term that the master will indemnify the servant from liability arising out of an unlawful enterprise upon which he has been required to embark without knowing it was unlawful'. Compare with the case below:

Box 6.8 Case: Lister v Romford and Cold Storage Co. Ltd. [1957] AC 555 at 595

In this case, a truck driver while in the course of his employment as a truck driver negligently injured his father who was also an employee of the same company. The father successfully sued the employer based on the vicarious liability principle. The employer's insurers, in turn, sued the driver in his capacity as joint wrongdoer and for breaching an implied term of the contract of employment which requires of him a duty to take reasonable care in the execution of his duties.

The Crown Proceedings Act 1947, which came into force in 1948, made the National Health Service, as the largest employer of nurses and provider of care through the healthcare trusts, open to civil litigation. In the event of a patient sustaining injury through negligence of employees of the crown, government ministers or healthcare trusts or health boards as employees of the crown may now be held criminally and civilly liable:

(1) Subject to the provisions of this Act, the Crown shall be subject to all those liabilities in tort to which, if it were a private person of full age and capacity, it would be subject: –
    (a) in respect of torts committed by its servants or agents;
    (b) in respect of any breach of those duties which a person owes to his servants or agents at common law by reason of being their employer;

There are, nevertheless, a few exceptions; the royal mint and judges who are under qualified privilege are immune from criminal prosecution. Other exceptions are members of Parliament under parliamentary privilege, who are also immune from prosecution. The National Health Service and Community Care Act 1990 also states on 'crown immunity' that

1) the Subject to the following provisions of this section, on and after the day appointed for the coming into force of this subsection, no health service body shall be regarded as the servant or agent of the Crown or as enjoying any status, immunity or privilege of the Crown ... no health service body shall be regarded as the servant or agent of the Crown or as enjoying any status, immunity or privilege of the Crown.
                    (Section 60, NHS and Community Care Act 1990 [c. 19])

The Health and Safety at Work Act 1974, introduced a new statutory duty of care (of health and safety) on trusts, trust boards and health providers as organizations has been created, making healthcare providers both criminally and civilly liable for the actions or omissions of the organization as a whole. If a healthcare worker fails to follow an employer's policy or procedure, then they may also find themselves jointly or singly liable for any negligent actions. nurses should have indemnity cover in the event of litigation. This would be provided by membership of a union.

The Health and Safety at Work Act 1974 may now be used for prosecuting and imposing fines and criminal prosecution by the Health and Safety Executive (HSE), as government watchdog. The HSE issues guidelines on health and safety and provides both informal and formal advice on health and safety. They may also issue improvement or enforcement notices with fines. Occasionally they may also serve a prohibition notice, stopping a business from operating. This followed several incidents of food poisoning in national Health Service (NHS) establishments. In 2012, 585 cases were prosecuted by the HSE, securing a conviction of 537 (92 per cent) (HSE, 2013) for all the United Kingdom. Under the Health and Safety (Offences) Act 2008, magistrate courts may impose a maximum fine of £20,000 for breaches of health and safety plus compensation for the victim as well as costs. Because the damages awarded in a criminal health and safety case are relatively small (as low as £5,000), the victim may wish to pursue civil litigation for compensation for harm, with potentially more damages.

The government vision had drawn up the white paper *The New NHS: Modern, Dependable* (DoH, 1997) which proposed a statutory duty for chief executives of healthcare organizations to implement systems of clinical governance to ensure good quality care. This change has seen a rise in litigation in clinical negligence actions:

12H –

(1) it shall be the duty of each Health Board, Special Health Board and NHS trust and of the Agency to put and keep in place arrangements for the purpose of monitoring and improving the quality of health care which it provides to individuals.
(2) The reference in subsection (1) to health care which a body there mentioned provides to individuals includes health care which the body provides jointly with another person to individuals.
(3) In this section 'health care' means services for or in connection with the prevention, diagnosis or treatment of illness.

(Section 51 of Health Act 1999)

On Individual Insurance, the NMC now requires this since 2014. This is especially the case for autonomous practitioners.

Appropriate cover is an indemnity arrangement which is appropriate to your role and scope of practice and its risks. The cover must be intended to be sufficient to meet an award of damages if a successful claim is made against you.

(www.nmc-uk.org/indemnity)

If a service user is harmed, under Health and Safety, they have a right to litigate and seek damages in compensation. There is no appeal if patients are unhappy with a Hand Safety award decision. The alternative is a claim in tort, the victim can institute legal proceedings unless they have accepted an out-of-court settlement, which may be preferable due to the practical difficulties in passing through the litigation hurdles of establishing a claim for negligence as well as the length of time this may take (see Chapter 2 above). Any claims should be within three years of the date of the civil wrong unless this is extended to up to six years at the discretion of the court, under the Limitation Act 1980 or the Prescription and Limitation (Scotland) Act 1973. Under the Employers Liability (Compulsory Insurance) Acts 1969 and 1998 (as amended by the Employers' Liability (Compulsory Insurance) (Amendment) Regulations 2004), employers are required to have insurance cover, in the event of claims. Since 1995, the national Health Service Clinical Negligence Scheme for Trusts (CNST) has been established as the body responsible for an 'insurance policy' for any NHS clinical negligence claims. The Scheme applies to any liability in tort owed by a member to a third party with respect to or consequent upon personal injury or loss arising out of or in connection with any breach of a duty of care owed by that body to any person in connection with the diagnosis of any illness, or the care or treatment of any patient, in consequence of any act or omission to act on the part of a person employed or engaged by a member in connection with any relevant function of that member (National Health Service [Clinical Negligence Scheme] NHS Resolution). Since April 2019, there has been a new Clinical Negligence Scheme for General Practice (CNSGP), a state-backed indemnity Scheme for general practice.

Occupier's liability – people on premises

Most care is provided in designated buildings, but the occupier's duty of care also extends to vehicles such as ambulances where care may be provided. The duty of care in this area comes under what is known as 'strict ability'. The aim is to provide maximum possible protection for a 'visitor'. This includes any person present on the premises who may suffer harm.

Subject to land law, an occupier is any person who has possession of premises and owns them (in the tenancy sense) and has control of activities in a building or vessel. The term 'premises' should be construed in its broadest sense, to include vehicles; for example, a patient being transported in an ambulance which is not roadworthy should be protected (from injury) by the law. The rationale behind this legislation means that any persons entering premises should be protected from any danger whether this is an obvious or latent defect which may harm them. The common law creates a duty of care to ensure that they are protected. Examples of unsafe premises are slips, trips and falls. There are two categories of persons who can be present on premises, categorized respectively as visitors and trespassers as recognized by the following pieces of legislation that deal in this area:

1. Occupier's Liability Act 1957 (OLA 1957)
2. Occupier's Liability Act 1984 (OLA 1984)

The aim of the first statute is to create a 'common law duty of care' for the occupier to avoid harm toward persons entering premises. The second statute, however, modified this requirement for the purpose of limiting liability where trespassers are concerned.

Occupier's liability act 1957

A 'visitor' is anyone who enters any premises for a legitimate purpose. This permission to be on premises is either explicit or implied. The OLA 1957 recognizes the 'common duty of care' to visitors (Section 2(2) of OLA 1957). This duty is to provide reasonable safety (Elliott and Quinn, 2019). As invitees include visitors who are legitimately on premises, such as patients, their visitors, as well as the nurse, these individuals should all be clearly owed a duty of care. The law expects higher standards of care as illustrated in the following case involving children, who are assumed to be less careful than adults.

Box 6.9 Case: Glasgow Corporation v Taylor [1922] 1 AC 44, 61

A seven-year-old child died after eating poisonous berries from a bush in a park owned by the corporation. The court considered that tempting to children since they looked like cherries.

Held: The corporation had breached their duty of care.

Subject to this statute, if injury is established, the duty of care arises on a 'strict liability' basis, with no requirement on the part of the victim to prove fault. This means that the law gives a victim additional protection by presuming absolute or strict liability on the part of the occupier of a building.

Occupier's liability act 1984

While the 1957 Act protects only invited persons or those who are implicitly or explicitly invited by the occupier, in contrast, the Occupier's Liability Act 1984 (OLA) statute may afford protection to those who are uninvited or trespassers, such as children, who may wander onto premises. This statute requires no strict liability unless it can be proved that the occupier (or owner of the premises) knows of or is aware of the danger, in which case the law expects them to afford reasonable protection to the trespasser. This principle is established in the following case:

Box 6.10 Case: White v St Albans City [1990] CA, reported in The Times, 12 March 1990

The claimant fell down a trench and sustained injury after he had taken a shortcut across council-owned land in order to access a car park. The land was privately owned, and surrounded by a fence, and there was no evidence that the council was aware of its use as a shortcut.

Held: The court of appeal held on evidence that the council had taken reasonable care and was therefore not liable.

As an occupier of premises, a hospital providing health care is entitled in civil law to put forward certain defences to a claim for damages in tort for personal injury (e.g. 'contribution'), which means that any damages awarded may be reduced in proportion to a victim's contribution. Another example of a defence is under the *volenti non fit injuria* principle (Section 2(5) of the 1957 Act), which means that 'the victim knowingly undertook the risk'. If the court finds for the defendant, it may in such cases reduce the level of damages awarded. A hospital (as occupier) may put up warning signs pointing out the danger or hazard but cannot exclude liability under any terms of contract (Section 2(3) of the Unfair Contract Terms Act 1979) in the event of another person being injured or killed.

Health and Safety is an established employment law concept with statutory criminal liability, with its main objective as safeguarding patients, as well as staff and visitors. Most care is provided in designated buildings, but the occupier's duty of care also extends to vehicles such as ambulances where care may be provided. The duty of care in this area comes under what is known as 'strict ability'. The aim is to provide maximum possible protection for a 'visitor'. This includes any person present on the premises who may suffer harm. A victim does not need to prove negligence on the part of the owner of a building.

Safe medicines management and administration

Medicine is an important area for safety due to the potential risk. The most frequently reported types of medication incidents involve wrong dose, omitted or delayed medicines or wrong medicine Over 90 per cent of incidents reported are associated with no harm or low harm (National Patient Safety Agency (NPSA), 2013). A National Framework for Reporting and Learning from Serious Incidents Requiring Investigation. The framework is also the first stage in the development of a consolidated Serious Incident framework NHS (2015).

It is therefore important that nurses ensure the safekeeping and administration of medications. In some cases, the fact senior nurses may also prescribe medicines may allow continuity and better monitoring for the patient.

- Two examples of legislation in this area include the following:
- Medicines Act 1986, which covers key issues such as the prescription, storage and dispensing and administration of medications;
- Misuse of Drugs Act 1973, which regulates the classification and storage of controlled drugs.

Medicine administration involves risk assessment and management in several stages including the following stages:

- A prescriber should consider the pharmacokinetics, what effect the medication has on the body, and the pharmacodynamics, how the body reacts to the medication. This may be positive or negative. Adverse reactions may result in a percentage of people. A prescriber must ensure the correct medication dose and the most effective route. They may also need to check the physical condition, age and weight of the patient, as well as other medications. This may cause interaction especially for patients with polypharmacy.
- Prescribing has been traditionally the domain of medical professionals such as the doctor or dentist, though with extended practice, senior nurses and pharmacists who have undergone appropriate training can prescribe.
- The pharmacist's main role is to dispense medication, though some may also be prescribers. The level of safety expected of pharmacists when dispensing medications to hospitals is the same expected of them when supplying and dispensing in the community to individuals.
- The next stage involves preparation of medication, for example, intravenous fluids. It is important on grounds of safety that manufacturers' and prescribers' instructions are followed accurately.
- A nurse administering medication must ensure the accuracy as well as the appropriate route and method. If patients are self-administering medication, they should have been risk assessed as competent. If the nurse administers medication, they must ensure the completion of this stage and not rely on others, without checking. An accurate record should be made contemporaneously (Royal Pharmaceutical Society, Royal College of Nursing, 2019).

The last import stage is the need to monitor the patient after the medication is given in case of adverse reactions. Furthermore, it is clear that

> Millions of medicines are prescribed in the community and in hospitals across England and Wales each day – the majority of these are delivered correctly and do exactly what they are meant to do. However, when an incident does occur, it is vital we learn from this to ensure patients are not harmed.
>
> (Fletcher, 2009, chief executive, NPSA, in Tackling Medication Incidents and Increasing Patient Safety, NPSA)

The NHS Improvement works closely with the Medicines Healthcare Regulatory Authority (MHRA) in monitoring standards. The MRHA is authorized by Directive 2001/83/EC relating to medicinal products for human use, amended by Directives 2002/98/EC, 2003/63/EC, 2004/24/EC and 2004/27/EC. They concluded,

> Safety, quality and efficacy are the only criteria on which legislation to control human medicines is founded. It is the responsibility of the MHRA and the expert advisory bodies set up by the Medicines Act to ensure that the sometimes difficult balance between safety and effectiveness is achieved. MHRA experts assess all applications for new medicines to ensure they meet the required standards. This is followed up by a system of inspection and testing which continues throughout the lifetime of the medicine. Safety monitoring is also continuous and the MHRA also ensures that doctors and patients receive up-to-date and accurate information about their medicines. This is achieved by ensuring that product labels, leaflets, prescribing information and advertising meet the required standards laid down by the Regulations.
>
> (MRHA, 2013)

Other relevant requirements include the ability for the reader to identify the prescriber and the person who administers medication, so it is important that records are clearly identifiable and signed with an identifiable designation, in the case of written records (NMC, 2018). Records may also be used by employers and defence lawyers as evidence in a court of law as well as by a litigant patient's counsel. The courts are likely to take the view that if something is not written down, then it did not happen, as verbal accounts of events are unreliable, especially with passage of time due to the failing human memory – events simply become more blurred or individuals may be making them up.

Conclusion

Bioethical principles should underpin clinical practice. This means that should a nurse's actions be called to account, the courts will look sympathetically toward a defendant nurse if they can demonstrate that they acted as a reasonable person following policy and procedures on patient safety. There may, of course, be a few unmanageable risks; it is a question of level of risk. The starting point for the nurse should be to understand the relevance of NMC Code of Professional Conduct (2018) in setting professional standards. It is also important to be aware of the impact of the law, national policy on health and safety legislation which should underpin decision-making in making clinical judgements. Any breach of professional regulations (misconduct) may also have legal consequences. On the other hand, ethical dilemmas may arise in practice; though this does not necessarily have legal or professional implications, it is almost certain that unethical conduct will breach other inextricable aspects of care. An ethical dilemma therefore presents challenges for the nurse while working in partnership with the patient, family member, carers and multi-disciplinary team as well as in collaboration with other agencies. In response to a complaint, a nurse would need to demonstrate that the care they gave was not only in the patient's best interests but that expected of a reasonable competent clinician who professes to have that skill (the Bolam Test). This should consider following guidelines as well as evidence-based practice for ensuring safety within the clinical working environment.

References

Adair J. *The skills of leadership.* Aldershot: Gower Publishing Company Limited, 1984.

Aiken LH, Clarke, Sloane DM, Sochalski J and Silber JH. Hospital nurse staffing and patient, 2002 mortality, nurse burnout, and job dissatisfaction. *JAMA* 2002; 288: 1987–93.

Bolam v Friern Hospital Management Committee [1957] 1 WLR 582.

Consumer Protection Act 1987 (Product Liability) (Modification) Order 2000.

Consumer Protection Act 1987 (Product Liability) (Modification) (Scotland) Order 2001.

Control of Substances Hazardous to Health Regulations (COSHH) 1999. Section 17.

Croner CCH Group. *Health and safety A–Z, essentials.* Kingston upon Thames: Croner CH Group, 2002.

DH (2003) NHS confidentiality code of practice. Available online at: www.doh.gov.uk (accessed on 1st February 2019).

DoH. HSC 1998/89, implementing the recommendations of the Caldicott Report, 1988.

DoH. *The protection and use of patient information.* HSG (96)18. Department of Health, 1996.

DoH. *Getting ahead of the curve: A strategy for combating infectious diseases.* A report by the chief medical officer. London: Crown, 2002.

DoH. *The Caldicott report* (1997) Available online at: www.doh.gov.uk (accessed on 3rd November 2019).

Donoghue v Stevenson [1932] UKHL 100.

EC Directive 85/374*l*.

EC Directive 85/374/EEC.

EC Directive 2002/98*l*.

EC Directive 2003/63*l*.

EC Directive 2004/24/EC.

EC Directive 2004/27/EC.

Elliott C and Quinn F. *Tort Law*, 12th ed. Harlow: Person Longman, 2019.

Francis R (2013) *Report of the Mid Staffordshire NHS Foundation Trust public inquiry.* London: The Stationery office. Available online at: tinyurl.com/HMSO-Francis2.

Glasgow Corporation v Taylor [1922] 1 AC 44, 61.

Health and Safety Executive (2013) Hospital trust improves floor cleaning after a slip. Available online at: http://www.hse.gov.uk/slips/experience/floorcleaning.htm (accessed on 2nd September).

Health and Safety Executive (2018/19) Available online at: http://www.hse.gov.uk/statistics/index.htm (accessed on 3rd June 2018).

Health and Safety Executive. Available online at: http://www.hse.gov.uk/coshh/ (accessed July 2010).

Health and Safety Executive (2001) Guidance on manual handling in people's home. Available online at: http://www.hse.gov.uk (accessed on 2nd June 2019).

Health and Safety Executive (2013) *Moving and handling in health and social care.* Available online at: http://www.hse.gov.uk (accessed on 14th October 2019).

Health and Safety (Consultation with Employees) Regulations 1996.

Health and Safety at Work Act 1974 Section 2, 2 (1) & 7.

Houses of Parliament Parliamentary Office (2017) UK Trends in Infectious Disease, Number 545 January 2017.

Human Rights Act 1998 Article 4 & 14.

Hunt G. *Freedom to care.* Available online at: https://www.freedom2care.org/ (accessed on 9th January 2006).

International Council of nurses. The ICN code of ethics for nurses. Available online at: https://www.icn.ch/sites/default/files/inline-files/2012_ICN_Codeofethicsfornurses_%20eng.pdf (accessed on 22nd June 2019).

Kingsfund, High quality care for all: NHS next stage review final report. Department of Health. 2008, p. 47. Available online at: https://www.kingsfund.org.uk/sites/default/files/briefing-high-quality-care-for-all-jo-maybin-ruth-thorlby-kings-fund-july-2008.pdf (accessed on 20th December 2019).

Liberty Protection Safeguards (2019).

Lister and Others v Hall [2001] UKHL 22.

Lister v Romford and Cold Storage Co. Ltd. [1957] AC 555 at 595.

Mandelstam M. *Quick guide to community care practice and the law.* Revised 6th ed. London: Jessica Kingsley, 2017.

Manual Handling Operations Regulations: Lifting Operations and Lifting Equipment Regulations 1998.

Manual Handling Operations Regulations (MHOR) 1992.

Medicines Act 1986.

MHRA. (2013) How we regulate medicines. Available online at: http://www.mhra.gov.uk/how-weregulate/Medicines/ (accessed on 15th July 2019).

Misuse of Drugs Act 1973.

NPSA (2008) A risk matrix for risk managers. Available online at: https://www.neas.nhs.uk/media/118673/foi.16.170_-_risk_matrix_for_risk_managers_v91.pdf.

National Patient Safety Agency (NPSA), 2013 incidents p. 19.

Needleman J and Buerhaus P. International Journal for Quality in Health Care. *Nurse staffing and patient safety: Current knowledge and implications for action.* 2003.

NHS Constitution (2015) Available online at: https://www.gov.uk/government/publications/the-nhs-constitution-for-england (Accessed on 1st October 2019).

NHS Improvement (2015) Serious Incident Framework. Available online at: https://improvement.nhs.uk/documents/954/Serious_Incident_framework_NHS_England_pdf (accessed on 20th November 2019).

NICE (2015) National Institute for Health and Care Excellence, health and social care directorate quality standards and indicators briefing paper. Available online at: https://www.nice.org.uk/guidance/qs113/documents/healthcareassociated-infections-qs-briefing-paper2 (Accessed on 22nd December 2019).

Nightingale F (1820–1910). Notes on nursing: What nursing is, what nursing is not. Philadelphia, London, Montreal: J.B. Lippincott Co. 1946 Reprint. First published London, 1859: Harrison & Sons. Retrieved 6 July 2010.

NPSA. Available online at: http://www.nrls.npsa.nhs.uk/ (accessed on 1st July 2019).

Nursing and Midwifery Code of Conduct (2018) Available online at: https://www.nmc.org.uk/standards/code/ (accessed on 30th May 2019).

Occupier's Liability Act 1957 Section 2 (5).

Occupier's Liability Act 1984.

Office of National Statistics (ONS) Available online at: http://www.ons.gov.uk/ons/index.html (accessed on 22nd July 2019).

Patients' Charter (1992) Available online at: https://publications.parliament.uk/pa/cm199192/cmhansrd/1991-11-05/Orals-1.html (accessed on 4th November 2019).

Phillips G and Scott K. *Employment law.* Guildford: College of Law Publishing, 2008.

Report of the Public Inquiry into children's heart surgery at the Bristol Royal Infirmary 1984–1995, Learning from Bristol (2001).

Reporting of Injuries, Disease and Dangerous Occurrences Regulations 1995.

Reporting of Injuries, Disease and Dangerous Occurrences (RIDDOR) Regulations 2013.

Ridley J. *Health and safety in brief,* 4th ed. Burlington: Butterworth Heinemann, 2008.

Royal College of nursing. *RCN code of practice for patient handling.* London: RCN Publication, 2002.

Royal Pharmaceutical Society, RCN (2019) Professional Guidance on the Administration of Medicines in Healthcare Settings.

Royal Pharmaceutical Society, Royal College of Nursing 2019.

Safety and Safety Committees Regulations 1977.

Safety Representatives and Safety Committees Regulations 1977.

Selwyn N. *Law of employment,* 16th ed. London: Butterworth, 2011.

Unfair Contract Terms Act 1977 Sections. 2(3), 16.

UNISON. Hospital contract cleaning and infection control (2004) Available online at: https://pdfs.semanticscholar.org/cde2/93ab760261a8c10d69a203e00184661218d2.pdf (accessed on 10th July 2019).

Weddall v Barchester Healthcare Ltd [2012] EWCA Civ 25.

White v St Albans City [1990] CA, reported in *The Times,* 12 March 1990.

Vulnerable adults, elder abuse

Chapter outline

Introduction
Background, adults at risk, the framework
Key theories and abuse
Human rights and abuse
Safeguarding and interventions
Criminal law sanctions
Civil law remedies
Service users with mental health needs
Interagency working and abuse
Conclusion

Introduction

The main subject matter for this chapter is vulnerable adults, focussing on older people who may fall victims to abuse. The principles herein may be applicable to any vulnerable group. Vulnerability is associated to most people with health and social care needs. There are similarities in cases of child abuse, the Children Acts 1989 and 2004 have put in place effective measures for protection, although cases like that of Victoria Climbié (from children's perspective) have shown how ineffective the system can be if healthcare professionals fail to intervene and safeguard victims. The Children Act 1989, the Children (Scotland) Act 1995 and the Children Act 2004 have been appropriate responses in providing clear rules on safeguarding the child's best interests. The 2004 Act statute also establishes the role of a national children's champion who focusses on national issues related to child abuse (see Chapter 3). There has been, however, no such specific provision for the protection of older people who may fall victim to abuse with a need of a clear definition of who is a vulnerable adult. This chapter focusses on the older patient, although the principles are equally applicable to other groups of victims of abuse such as children and all other groups of vulnerable adults

Background, adults at risk, the framework

A person aged 18 years or over who is or may need community care services by reason of mental or other disability, age or illness; and who is or may be unable to take care of him or herself, or unable to protect him or herself against significant harm or exploitation, Who Decides, 1997, Lord Chancellor's Department and, No Secrets, 2000, Department of Health Guidance.

The National Service Framework for Older People (2001) classified people over the age of 65 as older people. The WHO (World Health Organization) have defined an 'older person' as someone 'whose age has passed the median life expectancy at birth', which in the UK is currently 81.2 for men and women combined' (Centre for Policy on Ageing, 2009).

While it is not necessarily the case that all older people are vulnerable, they do represent the largest proportion of clientele receiving care within the NHS and private healthcare providers. With age, increases the likelihood of vulnerability increases as we become more dependent physically and psychologically. In different types of abusive situations, there is a common element – a breach of trust. The general principles are applicable to any type of abuse in respect of all client groups receiving health and/ or social care. Depending on a given situation, interventions to deal with the problem will be different. It is always difficult to establish the extent of any abuse due to possible underreporting as well as lack of evidence in support of any complaints as abuse may be perpetrated behind closed doors.

Box 7.1 Thinking point

1   What are the human rights linked to elder abuse?
2   What are the 'tell-tell' signs of abuse?
3   Following your local policy, what interventions should be applied in order to safe-guard vulnerable older people who may be at risk?

When abuse involves a vulnerable person, it could prove to be more difficult to manage if the abuser is a carer or a close family member, currently caring for the victim. Available responses are through piecemeal legislation without specific safeguards as in child law. This may cause confusion and frustration not only in the minds of the victims and their advocates but also in that of the perpetrator, who may not be aware that their action may be tantamount to abuse. An established definition of elder abuse is:

> A single or repeated act or appropriate action occurring within a relationship where there is an expectation of trust which causes harm or distress to an older (dependent) person.
>
> (Action on Elder Abuse, 1995)

The term 'elder abuse' has been in use for some time in the United States but is relatively new in the UK (Bennett and Kingston (1995) are accredited with adopting its use). There may be a preference for the term 'maltreatment' or 'mistreatment' to include both 'abuse' and 'neglect'. The latter is just as bad despite the passive element of 'doing nothing'. The effect may still be abuse. It has been suggested that up to 2.6 per cent of people aged 66 and over living in private households admitted having experienced mistreatment by a carer, including family members, a close friend or a care worker (O'Keeffe et al., 2007).

The debate on elder abuse has rekindled issues on the welfare and rights of people over the age of 65, especially those who may be dependent for their care and are therefore vulnerable and open to abuse. Abuse may take place either in the victim's own home or in an institution providing care such as a residential care home or hospital. It is possible that some abuse may remain unreported due to the secretive nature of abuse – behind closed doors. Abuse involves violation of an individual's human rights by any other person or persons covering a broad range of situations. This breach may be covered by law – the European Convention on Human Rights 1950 under Articles 3 and 17, also Schedule 1 Human Rights Act 1998, although the numbers of cases which have gone to law in this area are limited. The ONS (2019) showed that 'women were around twice as likely to have experienced domestic abuse than men (7.9% compared with 4.2%)'.

Given the definition of abuse in the government paper Protection of Vulnerable Adults (POVA) 2000, it is possible to conceive of victims of elder abuse as only those who are dependent on another for their care (POVA, 2000). In fact, any older person may be subject to abuse without the 'dependency' requirement. The emphasis should therefore be on 'vulnerability' instead.

Key theories and abuse

Criminological theories attempt to offer some explanations on why some perpetrators become violent and abusive and why some victims accept abuse as part and parcel of life. There is a link between the term 'abuse' and its generic term 'violence'. The difference is that violence may take place between strangers, while abuse occurs within a trusting relationship between the abuser and the victim. In the latter situation there is a breach of trust and there may be fear and dependency from the victim's perspective. Often, deception is involved, but it is unlikely that there is collusion on the part of the victim. Usually there is no choice in the outcome from the view of the victim as they may have been let down by those they trusted. A further element is the imbalance of power between the abuser and the victim. This is the position in which older people that are vulnerable find themselves. Only the main theories are included here in the attempt to explain why violence is perpetrated, with vulnerable people in general as well as the elderly in particular at the receiving end.

Biological and psychological theories

These two terms are related and have been put forward to explain how biological or psychological makeup may affect the behaviour of a potential abuser. The main theories aim to link behaviour with genetic traits, which are thought to cause a predisposition toward violent behaviour. It has been suggested that some violent men possess an extra male Y chromosome (Herrnstein and Murray, 1994). For some individuals this may include paranoia, which is supposedly determined by abnormalities in the chromosomes relating to the XXY and XYY factors (Williams, 2012). This condition is treatable through hormonal therapy. From the above, there has been a suggestion of a link to criminality for the XYY factor, which is the syndrome where the extra male chromosome is present, and another view is 'that chromosome abnormality and criminality are not closely related, and more significantly, if general explanations are wanted, the incidence of XXY and XYY males is so rare as to be of little practical significance' (Williams, 2012, p. 147).

The so-called 'naturalistic studies' have suggested that the children of criminals are more likely to become criminals themselves in later life, as a 'natural tendency' (Fitzgerald et al., 1981, p. 371). Eysenck (1977), however, has explained this behaviour as merely conditioned responses, which are achieved through operant conditioning, in the Pavlovian sense.

Cultural and social learning theories

These theories attribute the apparently higher level of domestic violence and abuse of wives and children in some cultures than in others to a learned process of the adoption of certain norms of behaviour from an early age. Some authorities suggest that society sets norms which become accepted and standard for that individual society. These norms may be enacted into law (Williams, 2012). The values of a society in how it relates to the treatment of women seem to be based on the acceptance of certain norms of behaviour. The cultural basis of the prevalence of violence only serves to explain the existence of accepted standards of behaviour in any given situation. This does not necessarily support the myth that some ethnic groups are more violent than others toward their female partners. Some studies have shown that cultural behaviour is passed on from generation to generation. On people in relationships, Hertzberger (1996, p. 109) concluded that the 'majority of abusive spouses and their victims are more likely to have a history of abuse by their parents'. These norms are supposed to reinforce the concept of a male-dominated society, with women, children and the elderly as victims, and this is unfortunate as it may give the impression that most abusers are male. It is not possible to prove conclusively that culture, whether racial, geographical or social class related, per se, is responsible for domestic violence and the abuse of vulnerable people, such as the elderly. It is possible that partner abuse may be used as a tool to exercise control and subjugate the weaker person. Other attempts to explain violence in the family context have been based on social learning. Some base domestic violence and cultural abuse on the 'subculture of violence', by attributing it to men's 'susceptibility', which Curtis (1975) put down to racism and economic oppression.

The Social Learning theory of Albert Bandura (1977) is one of the most fascinating contributions from behaviourists who have made an important contribution to the debate on learned criminal behaviour which is said to result in abuse of elderly persons by their own children, if the latter have been brought up previously experiencing a culture of abuse. The basis of this theory is that behaviour is learnt through observation of violent behaviour. This could be explained by a negative effect not only from the family, but also from society as a whole (which may be seen as uncaring toward its older persons) as well as media sources such as television and press; 'children and adults acquire attitudes, emotional responses and new styles of conduct through filmed television modelling' (Bandura, 1977, p. 39). This process is called 'modelling'. This would explain the future presence of criminal or violence behaviour in individuals who have been exposed to violence as children. As to the question why there are more men abusers and more female victims, Bandura (1977) suggests that 'boys more readily imitate the aggression they observe in others ... girls in contrast refrain from imitating, unless explicitly informed that aggressive behaviour is acceptable' (cited in Hertzberger, 1996, p. 118). Other factors, for example, alcohol and drug abuse, can be contributory to violence and elder abuse, and may sometimes be used as an excuse. Studies have shown a correlation between alcohol and substances and criminal behaviour in the home by someone who already has a criminal propensity (Williams, 2012). Alcohol not only acts as a depressant but may also remove inhibitions, thus making it easier for a carer of an elderly person who has experienced pent-up feelings of stress to be more aggressive and abusive. It is possible that alcohol will be used as an excuse for violence. There may very well be other related causes, such as 'paying back' old scores to a previously abusive parent or spouse for whose care they may be responsible.

The feminist perspective – learned helplessness

Feminist theories generally attribute the trend toward violence as evidence of the inequality between men and women. This view is consistent with other factors such as economic dependence and the lower earning power of women, as well as a conflict of interests between spouses. These principles could apply to any relationships or equally to men who are subjected to abuse in their own homes by women. Some attribute the 'imbalance' between men and women to men's 'economic strength' and support in the home (Williams, 2012). The issue of dependence can limit the victim in the options available to them.

A survey of older people (Bennett, 2002) suggested that the only three broad areas they (as potential and actual victims) considered to amount to abuse were as follows:

- neglect – this may be caused by the victim themselves or may be a result of omissions of others;
- violation of human rights which may have legal as well as medical implications;
- deprivation of some privilege, which may include substitution of choices and decisions.

The above categories demonstrate that there are aspects of abuse that elderly people themselves may not consider to be abuse. Therefore, they may not feel it necessary to report the abuse and may consider it as their 'lot', an acceptable phenomenon (Bennett, 2002). Understanding classifications of abuse is important for healthcare professionals, so that they may appreciate the range of issues they may have to deal with. It is generally accepted that there are at least five types of abuse.

There is a consensus of other common classifications, which includes the following:

- Physical: This involves contact or battery, which may include inflicting physical harm such as restraining as well as the inappropriate administration of medications.
- Psychological: This would include swearing, threats of violence, insults, mental torture, humiliation, belittling someone and social isolation.
- Financial/property: This covers misappropriation of all forms of possessions belonging to an elderly person (see Chapter 8, 'Equality, diversity and inclusivity'). This would also include unauthorized and unexplained changes in wills and suspect bank or benefit transactions, often with the alleged abuser as beneficiary.
- Sexual: This involves rape, indecent assault, as well as any form of unwarranted touch and sexual innuendo (which is strictly speaking 'psychological'). Any sexual activity must be between consenting adults with mental capacity.

- Neglect: This may be carried out by others such as family members or carers, or self-inflicted. In some cases, the victim may not be aware of the resulting harm. It is nevertheless possible that self-neglect can take place, hence the need for a thorough investigation before accusing carers or family members. Should a person choose to take their own life, it is no longer a criminal offence for individuals to take their own life, under Section 2 of the Suicide Act 1961. It is nevertheless a crime to assist a suicide (see Chapter 9).

As well as a breach of duty of care, professionals may be found to be in breach of their duty of care when they fail to act to prevent abuse.

These categories are based on the British Geriatrics Society Classification (1998). The Department of Health (2001) in the government White Paper, No Secrets 2000 added another category, 'discriminatory abuse', to this (sometimes described as 'institutional'). This includes inadequate provisions for the elderly – it is questionable whether this should be a separate class (of ageism) from other grounds of discrimination such as religion, race, gender and sexual orientation (which may be recognized by the law). This may be related to a provision against age discrimination in employment law under the Employment Equality (Age) Regulations 2006. This is now covered by the Equality Act 2010.

An abuser could potentially be 'from a wide range of people including relatives and family members, as well as professional staff, paid care workers, volunteers, other service users, neighbours, friends and associates, people who deliberately exploit vulnerable people and strangers' {paragraph 2.10 of No Secrets (Department of Health, 2000)}.

It is important to consider the effectiveness of current responses in light of any staff training as well as clear guidelines, which should be proactive to minimize the risk of and counter abuse. However, these do not always offer sufficient protection to a victim. Abuse involving violent acts may amount to a criminal offence provided the elements of a crime, a guilty intention (*mens rea*) and a guilty act (*actus reus*) are proven. The Crown Prosecution Service under criminal law may prosecute the perpetrator. The difficulty is that the generic category of domestic abuse ranges from seemingly minor and harmless actions such as psychological abuse or harassment to those with more serious consequences like rape, serious assault or murder. It is possible that there may be 'window dressing' of the criminal act by using the term 'abuse' instead of more serious terminology. The difference between violence in general and elder abuse is the context within which it generally takes place. The British Crime Survey (1995) suggests that the highest number of assaults took place in the home, with '8 out of 10' victims of abuse being women (Donnellan, 2001, p. 2). Following several hospital episodes, signs of suspected abuse may be 'discovered' by a healthcare professional on admission assessments in accident and emergency departments, often unrelated to the apparent reason for admission:

> The signs of abuse are not always very obvious and may be uncovered secondary to other issues, perhaps when a client is admitted to care following alleged 'falls', clinical findings may not be consistent with the pre-admission history and the client's health status.
>
> (Fletcher and Buka, 1999, p. 155)

The main problem facing the healthcare professional in dealing with vulnerable adult abuse is that it is difficult to prove abuse and a victim may not wish to report it if this involves a close family member. Nevertheless, if they suspect abuse healthcare professionals are duty-bound to report it to other members of the multidisciplinary team. They must follow their own local guidelines on the process for reporting abuse. nurses may find themselves in a dilemma between the need for confidentiality and the necessity to breach this if their patient's safety is under threat (if a crime has been or is about to be committed), if disclosure is in the public interest, as required by statute or if ordered to disclose by a court of law (NMC Code of Conduct, 2018). The Caldicott principles provide further clarification in this area (Department of Health, 1997). Any disclosure of confidential information is subject to the Data Protection Act 1998.

Human rights and abuse

The European Convention on Human Rights 1950 became part of UK human rights law after the passing of the Human Rights Act 1998 (implemented in 2000). Under articles in Schedule 1, for example, Articles 3 and 17, a victim of abuse may take a public body such as a local authority or a healthcare trust to court. In dealing with them, the issue of abuse may not be resolved in the UK courts, and then an appeal is lodged to the European Court of Human Rights in Strasbourg. It also means that a victim may rely on the human rights legislation (in UK courts) without seeking redress from the European Court of Human Rights (Leach, 2017).

Although this was intended to enhance the rights of victims, the Articles of the European Convention on Human Rights 1950, do not go far enough as this is limited to abuse in a caring environment which is provided by a public body only. A victim of abuse who is in care provided by a private home may not rely on this legislation but instead pursue criminal and civil law. The Public Interest Disclosure Act 1998 should make it easier for healthcare workers who 'blow the whistle' on suspected abuse to be protected against victimization. In practice, victims may still be reluctant to go through the difficult procedures of having to give evidence against a loved one or losing them through imprisonment or enforced separation for their own protection. This has been recognized by the House of Commons (2004, paragraph 2) in the government's response to the recommendations and conclusions of the Health Select Committee's Inquiry into Elder Abuse.

Safeguarding and interventions

Before responding vigorously to allegations or apparent elder abuse, it may not in the first instance be necessary to warrant legal or other formal interventions, as things may not be what they seem (Buka and Sookhoo, 2006). There may also be a possibility of intervening informally (with limited evidence of abuse available) or reporting the matter to authorities in that a victim may through their own choice be considered responsible for their own self-neglect. It is important for clear guidelines in the clinical environment to minimize the risk to vulnerable older people. Doing nothing in the hope that things will resolve themselves is not an option as it is not hard to imagine the outcome of doing nothing. The problem is that without the active cooperation of a victim in any complaint investigation where there is suspected abuse, it may be difficult if not impossible to prosecute (Potter, 2017).

The Care Act 2014 creates a duty of local authorities to ensure safeguarding of adults at risk. Formal Interventions should always be through interdisciplinary settings so as to encourage a balanced and fairer outcome for both the patient and the alleged abuser, especially if this turns out to be unsubstantiated. Those involved should include multi-disciplinary healthcare professionals, as well as other interagency groups such as social services, the police and any local advocacy agencies (for example, Victim Support and Citizens Advice Bureau) to provide support. Cases of suspected abuse, in which there is evidence of a criminal act involving serious injury or death, must always be reported to the police in addition to following local procedure. Thereafter, the Crown Prosecution Service may decide to prosecute on the basis of the evidence or may not prosecute if it is not in the public interest to do so. Healthcare professionals may be reluctant to report the matter if there is any doubt, as they may be concerned about making the situation worse for the victim should their suspicions turn out to be ill founded. Abuse may amount to a criminal offence if the guilty intention is proven. Unintentional abuse also has adverse effects on an elderly victim, and depending on the degree of recklessness, if proven, could also be criminal negligence. Following several cases of elder abuse that have come to light, the government has responded with its White Paper No Secrets: The Protection of Vulnerable Adults (POVA, 2000).

Box 7.2 Thinking point: case study

Fitzgerald (the director of action on elder abuse) pointed out that many people would be familiar with the case of Victoria Climbié, but few knew about Margaret Panting, a 78-year-old woman from Sheffield who died after suffering 'unbelievable cruelty' while living with relatives. After her death in 2001, a post-mortem found 49 injuries on her body including cuts probably made by a razor blade and cigarette burns. She had moved from sheltered accommodation to her son-in-law's home – five weeks later she was dead, but as the cause of Margaret Panting's death could not be established, no one was ever charged. An inquest in 2002 recorded an open verdict (House of Commons, 2004).

The link between crime rates and elder abuse is not always easy to establish. An overview of related crime rates demonstrates that certain abuse-type crimes may also be on the increase (Home Office, 2003). Victim gender differences may also be indicative of the extent of the vulnerability of older people. Up to 20 per cent of persons over 85 years old attending A&E presented with trauma conditions, which could be linked to abuse (British Geriatrics Society Classification, 1998). These figures should, however, be treated with caution as they do not distinguish between other violent crimes and abuse (Home Office, 2003). For 2010–11, British Crime Survey (2011), 18.8 per cent of victims was aged over 65. 2018 figures also showed that three-quarters of domestic abuse-related offences the victim was female (75 per cent). For 'domestic abuse-related sexual offences the proportion of victims that were female was even higher, at 96%' Office of National Statistics (2019).

Box 7.3 Thinking point

M and S are daughters of John X, who has been deemed unable to cope on his own and required to be placed in a local authority nursing home three months after his wife's death (he had been the main carer for several years). The daughters live with their own families and visit their father in the residential home. Over the last two months they have noticed that he appears to be losing a lot of weight, and he has bruises on his upper arms. He is very sleepy whenever they visit; the staff nurse in charge says that he has been given (as required) zopiclone tablets as he keeps other residents awake. This makes him rather sleepy and unsteady during the day. They also noticed that he has a slight smell of urine and has not been bathed for several days, and they often have to ask the staff to change him. It seems to take a long time before he is changed, during visits. They (staff) say that the reason he is not attended to is that he refuses to get changed. He also appears to be frightened of one particular male agency carer. He begs his daughters to take him home.

They are worried about possible signs of abuse. Consider the case in light of your local policy or guidelines for managing elder abuse. What advice would you give in order to empower the victim?

Criminal law santions

Where there is evidence of a criminal act having taken place, the matter should be reported to the police. Based on the investigation and evidence, the Crown Prosecution Service may subsequently prosecute the abuser. It is necessary to prove the *mens rea* (a guilty mind) and *actus reus* (a guilty act). The burden of proof depends on the 'preponderance' or persuasiveness of evidence or how convincing the evidence may be, and this should go beyond reasonable doubt. More recent reports show that elder abuse is real.

Furthermore, this includes a broad group of vulnerable clients – anyone who has also been associated with a person who is receiving any form of health care is detained in a prison. This also includes remand centre, young offender institution, secure training centre or attendance centre or under the powers of the Immigration and Asylum Act 1999; is in contact with probation services. Every year, around 10 per cent of the population aged 65+ in the UK experiences some form of abuse. That's around 1 million people.

- 'Abuse' covers a range of criminal offences including physical and sexual assaults, financial crime such as theft and fraud, psychological torment and neglect.
- The number of calls received by Action on Elder Abuse's helpline from 1st May 2018-1st May 2019 was 8,530, a 4% increase on the previous year. Around 2,500 of these calls were taken on as "cases", investigated further by Action on Elder Abuse's dedicated team of staff and volunteers.
- The breakdown of cases by abuse type was as follows: Physical – 9%, Financial – 39%, Psychological – 34%, Neglect – 16%, Sexual – 1% (figures rounded to the nearest 1)

(HER Majesty's Inspectorate Constabulary and Fire and Rescue Services [HMICFRS])

An example is when there is a history of unexplained falls as well as suspicious behaviour. Some of the areas of law concerned with abuse include:

- Trespass to the person offences are covered by the Offences against the Person Act 1861. This involves physical contact which results in harm. Assault consists of verbal abuse only, and battery requires contact, from unwanted physical touch to inflicting actual harm, Scots law however defines both as assault. Unwanted treatment, while apparently acting 'in their best interests', is an example of the offence of battery. The patient has a right to privacy under Article 8 of the HRA 1998.
- Property offences are subject to Sections 1 and 15 of the Theft Act 1968, the Theft Act 1978 and the Theft (Amendment) Act 1996. This is a criminal offence of stealing goods (Section 1) or obtaining goods by deception under (Section 15).
- Sexual offences are mainly covered by the Sexual Offences Act 1984 and the Sexual Offences (Amendment) Act 2003. Should consent be given by a patient who lacks capacity, this is not valid, and an absolute offence where children are involved, and strict liability applies to non-consensual sext with a minor.
- Exclusion orders were introduced via Section 40A of the Powers of Criminal Courts (Sentencing) Act 2000, by Section 46 of the Criminal Justice and Courts Services Act 2000. The courts may ban a perpetrator from entering the premises (where an elder abuse victim is currently living) for up to two years.
- Antisocial behaviour orders (ASBOs) were introduced by the Crime and Disorder Act 1998. Subject to Section 1(a), an offender may be excluded (following a court order) from the alleged victim's place of residence.

A landlord, the police or local authority may also apply for the protection of the victim.

Civil law remedies

In addition, a victim can also seek remedies in the civil courts, that is damages in compensation for harm or personal injury, in conjunction with the above (criminal) measures. The victim may also apply for an injunction (which is a court order preventing conduct such as contact with the victim). Breach of such a court order will result in penalties such as imprisonment or a fine. The nature and levels of current legal responses may vary.

Personal injury claims

It is a long-established principle in negligence under Tort Law that a victim of harm resulting from another person' negligent actions is owed a duty of care, and they are entitled to damages for personal injury. This basic duty of care principle originated in *Donoghue v Stevenson [1932] AC 562,* and this law is further developed in *Caparo Industries v Dickman [1990] 2 AC 605* below. Care providers owe a duty of care not only to do good (benevolence), but also to avoid harm (nonmalevolence) to the persons who they provide care for. If the nurse as a carer is in breach of a duty of care, and the victim suffers harm (personal injury) as a result, the victim may be entitled to recover damages in compensation under tort law (or law of delict in Scotland).

In his famous judgement, in the same case, Lord Atkins established the duty of care principle:

> You must take reasonable care to avoid acts or omissions which you can reasonably foresee would be likely to injure your neighbour. Who, then, in law is my neighbour? The answer seems to be – persons who are so closely and directly affected by my act that I ought reasonably to have them in contemplation as being so affected when I am directing my mind to the acts or omissions which are called in question.
> (Lord Atkins, at p. 562, Donoghue v Stevenson [1932] AC 562)

A three-stage test for determining 'duty of care' has subsequently been applied by the courts in establishing the duty of care in the following case.

Box 7.4 Case: Caparo Industries v Dickman [1990] 2 AC 605

This was a landmark case where an auditor working for the defendants had compiled a report for Caparo, which showed that fidelity Co. was in profit. relying on this information Caparo bought shares. as it turned out, this was not the case and the plaintiff's shareholders lost money. The shareholders for Caparo sued the auditors who had compiled the report for negligence. it was held that there was no sufficient proximity of relationship between auditors and shareholders, thus setting out the three-stage test for duty of care:

1   whether there was foreseeability of harm,
2   whether there was a sufficient proximity of relationship between the parties,
3   whether it was just, fair and equitable for the court to impose a duty of care.

Furthermore, Section 46 of the Domestic Violence, Crime and Victims Act 2004 introduced a provision for the court to issue non-molestation orders for the protection of victims of abuse, provided the victim is living in the same household as the perpetrator of the abuse. There is law for protecting occupancy rights in Scotland in the form of the Matrimonial Homes (Family Protection) (Scotland) Act 1981. Such legislation may nevertheless still be breached, thus putting a victim of abuse at an even greater risk of retribution. Home Office (2011) sought to broaden the definition of domestic violence to include a broader group of clients, not simply adults in a relationship. Similarly, the duty of care is applied by the NMC Code (2018) through the requirement for the nurse to work with others to protect and promote the health and wellbeing of those in your care, their families and carers, and the wider community. This considers safety as on other key themes for safeguarding those at risk of harm.

Following several cases of domestic violence resulting in abuse and death of children, a new statute is in place which extends the offence of causing or allowing the death of a child or vulnerable adult in section 5 of the Domestic Violence, Crime and Victims Act 2004 Act ('the causing or allowing death offence') to cover causing or allowing serious physical harm (equivalent to grievous bodily harm) to a child or vulnerable adult ('the causing or allowing serious physical harm offence'). Domestic Violence, Crime and Victims (Amendment) Act 2012 (Commencement) Order 2012, SI 2012/1432 (c. 54)

Service users with mental health needs

It may be necessary to protect an at-risk elderly patient with mental health needs. In this case, compulsory orders are available for compulsory admission to a health-care facility for either a victim of abuse or the perpetrator (who has mental health needs) (Sections 2–5 of Mental Health Act 1983 or corresponding aspects of the Mental Health (Scotland) Act 1984). The mental health provisions may be used to protect the needs of individuals with mental health needs or those of their carers. For example, under Section 37 of the Mental Health Act 1983, the courts have powers to order hospital admission or guardianship. Alternatively, Section 43 of the same act defines the power of magistrates' courts to commit for a restriction order. Section 35 of the Mental Capacity Act 2005 provides additional protection for a vulnerable person who may be at risk to themselves or others, to have appointed another person (an independent mental capacity advocate) to look after their interests regarding consent to treatment, as they may be a victim of abuse. A community treatment order may be used if they need mental health treatment and may be at risk to others or of self-neglect under,

> The Mental Health Act 1983 S17 5)
> The relevant criteria are—
> (a) the patient is suffering from mental disorder of a nature or degree which makes it appropriate for him to receive medical treatment;
> (b) it is necessary for his health or safety or for the protection of other persons that he should receive such treatment;
> (c) subject to his being liable to be recalled as mentioned in paragraph (d) below, such treatment can be provided without his continuing to be detained in a hospital;

Mental capacity for the purposes of this statute includes both those who may have a temporary or permanent need. This power includes treatment as well as financial interests.

Interagency working in abuse cases

The following White Paper may be seriously flawed as it does not include those who may be victims of abuse but who do not receive community services (Parliamentary Select Committee on Health, February 2004). The aim of the above guidance is to bring together the various agencies responsible for the provision of care in the development of policies and procedures for the protection of vulnerable adults (including the elderly) from abuse. Health and social care providers benefit from working with all other agencies that may be involved in the care of the client.

Box 7.5 Thinking point

Mrs X is an 84-year-old lady who has been widowed for ten years, having had no children from her marriage. She has a niece who lives in Australia who is not able to visit and she last saw her at her uncle's funeral. Apart from that time, they never keep in

(continued)

(continued)

touch. Mrs X has become increasingly dependent on private carers as well as on her neighbours, Peter and his wife. He happens to be a qualified practicing adult nurse and his wife is a district healthcare assistant. They pop in every day and help with the shopping. Over the years Peter and his wife have become very close to Mrs X, who often treats them like family. She buys them and the children gifts for Christmas and birthdays. Peter also pays her bills and is an authorized signatory to Mrs X's bank accounts. She has three accounts but does not keep track of the large amounts in the bank since her husband died. she trusts Peter with her debit cards, and the district nurse who visits regularly suspects he might be withdrawing unauthorized large sums of money without Mrs X's knowledge. Peter has just bought himself a car paid for with Mrs X's (fraudulently obtained) money, but when confronted by the district nurse he says he bought the car (with Mrs X's permission) for taking Mrs X to the hospital for her appointments and a drive at the weekend, even though he also uses the car for personal use.

1   Consider what actions you would need to take in order to protect the patient.
2   Consider the NMC Code 2018 and consider what actions you may need to take.

The problem is that it is difficult to monitor what happens in individual private homes where most abuse is alleged to take place. In cases which may be drawn to their attention, social workers have at their disposal the powerful protective powers of Section 47 of the National Assistance Act 1948, to help them remove a victim of abuse to a place of safety if it is felt that they may be a danger to themselves or to others. In practice, this is difficult to enforce unless the victim has mental health needs. The Mental Capacity Act 2005 introduced additional guarantees of healthcare advocacy from April 2007, bringing English law into line with Scottish law, Mental Health (Care and Treatment) (Scotland) Act 2003. Informal arrangements alone may occasionally be adequate when the patient, family members or friends all agree that the multi-disciplinary team can pre-empt the situation by putting in place measures to minimize harm or remove a victim from the abusive environment. The following statute provides a welcome relief for a carer who may require respite and thus provide some relief.

A carer may request the local authority, before they make their decision as to whether the needs of the relevant person call for the provision of any services, to carry out an assessment of his ability to provide and to continue to provide care for the relevant person.

Section 1(b) of Carers (Recognition and Services) Act 1995
Safeguarding relates to the need to protect certain people who may be in vulnerable circumstances. These are people who may be at risk of abuse or neglect, due to the actions (or lack of action) of another person. In these cases, it is critical that services work together to identify people at risk and put in place interventions to help prevent abuse or neglect, and to protect people.
(Office of Public Guardian, Safeguarding Policy, 2013)

As part of the nurses' role in providing the best care in fulfilling their duty of care, they must ensure that especially where the client lacks capacity, they always act in the patient's best interests (Mental Capacity Act 2005). The NMC (2010) also requires the nurse to 'raise and escalate concerns'.

> If you witness or suspect there is a risk to the safety of people in your care and you consider that there is an immediate risk of harm, you should report your concerns without delay to the appropriate person or authority.
>
> (NMC, 2010, paragraph 6)

More therefore needs to be done to raise awareness and disclose, Public Interest Disclosure Act 1998.

Scotland provides free provision of personal care by local authorities, something which may be a contributing factor in lessening the chances of abuse by immediate family who are also carers (Community Care and Health (Scotland) Act 2002). Addressing assessments and safeguarding vulnerable adults should be inclusive and consider the informal carers who may themselves be vulnerable elders, some concerns and frustration about the limitation of the care framework in the UK (Bradley, 1996).

The Disclosure and Barring System, as provided by the Protection of Freedoms Act 2012, now aims to improve the vetting of abusers, actual or potential. It also merges the functions of the Criminal Records Bureau (CRB) and Independent Safeguarding Authority (ISA) (Home Office, 2013).

Conclusion

It is clear that as long as the causes for violent crimes exist, it is possible that vulnerable patients may be victims. Elder abuse, as any other type of abuse, tends to be subtle and secretive, and vulnerable older people may continue to suffer in secret, partly for fear of further victimization or because they feel disempowered. The importance of the healthcare professional's intervention is in being able to recognize the signs, being proactive and being able to prevent abuse from occurring.

As an integral part of a trusting relationship between nurse and patient, the patient (or client) should feel confident that the nurse (together with other carers and family members) is able to safeguard and afford them the protection and dignity they deserve and not victimize them. The NMC, (2018) Code requires the client's informed consent to treatment (in its widest context). Without obtaining (informed) consent, there may be overriding of the service user's rights. The nurse to 'identify' and minimize any risk to patients and clients. It is important for interagency communication to ensure that these rights are safeguarded and that preventative interventions are in place where there may be suspicion but insufficient evidence of abuse. The essential elements of establishing abuse should include evaluation and assessment.

It is important to recognize that abuse may come from the healthcare or care professionals who are supposed to protect the client. This is due to the dependency and the imbalance of power within the client-carer relationship. The nurse should be aware of the ethical values underpinning respect for their patient's values and ensure their right to autonomy or informed choice. Failure to consider this right may result in breach of human rights (Article 3 of the Human Rights Act 1998).

References

Action on Elder Abuse (AEA). Bulletin, May–June 1995.

Bandura A. *Social learning theory*. New York: General Learning Press, 1977.

Bennett G. Age and ageing. British Geriatric Society. 2002. Available online at: www.bgs.org.uk/Publications/age_ageing.htm (accessed 20th July 2013).

Bennett G and Kingston P. *Concepts, theories and interventions*. London: Chapman & Hall, 1995.

Bradley M. Caring for older people: Elder abuse. *BMJ* 1996; 313: 548–50. British Geriatrics Society (BGS). The abuse of older people. 1998. www.bgs.org.uk/ (accessed 29th August 2013).

British Crime Survey (1995).

British Crime Survey (2011).

British Geriatrics Society Classification (1998).

Buka P and Sookhoo D. Current legal responses to elder abuse. *International Journal of Older People Nursing* 2006; 1(4): 194–200.

Caparo Industries v Dickman [1990] 2 AC 605.

Care Act 2014.

Carers (Recognition and Services) Act 1995, S 1(b).

Centre for Policy on Ageing. *Ageism and age discrimination in primary and community health care in the United Kingdom*. London: Centre for Policy on Ageing, 2009.

Children Acts 1989 and 2004.

Children (Scotland) Act 1995.

Community Care and Health (Scotland) Act 2002.

Crime and Disorder Act 1998. Subject to Section 1(a).

Criminal Justice and Courts Services Act 2000, section 46.

Curtis L. *Violence, race and culture*. Lexington: Lexington Books, 1975.

Data Protection Act 1998.

Department of Health. Caldicott guardians. HSC 1999/012. 1997.

Department of Health. No secrets, guidance on developing and implementing multi-agency policies and procedures to protect vulnerable adults from abuse. HSC 2001/007: LAC (2001)12. London: Crown, 2000.

Domestic Violence, Crime and Victims Act 2004, sections 5, 46.

Domestic Violence, Crime and Victims (Amendment) Act 2012 (Commencement) Order 2012, SI 2012/1432 (c. 54).

Donnellan C. *Alcohol abuse issues*. Cambridge: Independence Educational Publishers, 2001.

Donoghue v Stevenson [1932] AC 562.

Employment Equality (Age) Regulations 2006.

Equality Act 2010.

European Convention on Human Rights 1950 under Articles 3 and 17.

Eysenck H. *Crime and personality*, 3rd ed. London: Routledge and Kegan Paul, 1977.

Fitzgerald M, McLennan G and Pawson J. *Crime and society: Readings in history and theory*. London: Open University Press, 1981.

Fletcher L and Buka P. *A legal framework for caring*. Basingstoke: Palgrave Macmillan, 1999.

Her Majesty's Inspectorate Constabulary and Fire and Rescue Services (HMICFRS). The poor relation the police and CPS response to crimes against older people July 2019. Available online at: www.justiceinspectorates.gov.uk/hmicfrs (accessed on 22nd October 2019).

Herrnstein RJ and Murray C. *The bell curve: Intelligence and class structure in American life*. New York: Free Press, 1994.

Hertzberger S. *Violence within the family. Sociology perspectives*. Oxford Social Psychology Series. Boulder: Westview Press, 1996.

HM Government. Abuse of vulnerable adults in England, 2011–12: Provisional report, experimental statistics. Available online at: www.data.gov.uk (accessed on 22nd August 2013).

Home Office. Crime in England and Wales. London: Home Office statistical bulletin. Crown, 2003. Available online at: https://www.legal-tools.org/doc/067b80/pdf/ (accessed on 3rd October 2019).

Home Office. Cross-government definition of domestic violence: A consultation. London: Home Office, 2011. Available online at: https://assets.publishing.service.gov.uk/government/uploads/system/uploads/attachment_data/file/116417/hosb1011.pdf (accessed on 2nd November 2019).

Home Office (2013) National archives, barring and disclosure service. http://webarchive.nationalarchives.gov.uk/20130107105354/http://homeoffice.gov.uk/agencies-public-bodies/dbs/ (accessed on the 30th August 2013).

House of Commons. The government's response to the recommendations and conclusions of the Health Select Committee. Crown, 2004.

Leach P. *Taking a case to the European Court of Human Rights*, 4th ed. Oxford: Oxford University Press, 2017.

Lord Chancellor's Department, No Secrets, 2000, No Secrets: Guidance on protecting vulnerable adults in care. Available online at: https://www.gov.uk/government/publications/no-secrets-guidance-on-protecting-vulnerable-adults-in-care (accessed on 3rd May 2019).

Matrimonial Homes (Family Protection) (Scotland) Act 1981.

Mental Capacity Act 2005.

Mental Health Act 1983, sections 2–5, sections 37, S17 5.

Mental Health (Scotland) Act 1984.

Mental Health (Care and Treatment) (Scotland) Act 2003.

National Assistance Act 1948, Section 47.

National Service Framework for Older People (2001).

NMC Code of Conduct, 2018.

NMC (2010) Raising and Escalating Concerns, Guidance for Nurses and Midwives, paragraph 6.

Office of National Statistics (2019) Domestic abuse in England and Wales: Year ending March 2018. Available online at: https://www.ons.gov.uk/peoplepopulationandcommunity/crimeandjustice/bulletins/domesticabuseinenglandandwales/yearendingmarch2018#domestic-abuse-recorded-by-the-police (accessed on 22nd July 2019).

Office of Public Guardian, Safeguarding Policy (2013) Available online at: http://www.justice.gov.uk/downloads/protecting-thevulnerable/mca/safeguarding-policy.pdf (accessed on 7th August 2019).

O'Keeffe M, Hills A, Doyle M, McCreadie C, Scholes S, Constantine R, Tinker A, Jill Manthorpe Biggs S, and Erens B. UK Study of Abuse and Neglect of Older People Prevalence Survey Report, National Centre for Social Research and King's College London, 2007. Available online at: http://www.natcen.ac.uk/media/308684/p2512-uk-elder-abuse-final-for-circulation.pdf (assessed on 20th April 2020).

Parliamentary Select Committee on Health (February 2004) Available online at: https://publications.parliament.uk/pa/cm200304/cmselect/cmhealth/cmhealth.htm (accessed on 18th October 2019).

Potter J. Behind closed doors: Abuse of the elderly patient. *Nursing in Practice* 2017; 14: 21–23.

Powers of Criminal Courts (Sentencing) Act 2000 Public Interest Disclosure Act 1998.

Protection of Freedoms Act 2012.

Sexual Offences Act 1984.

Sexual Offences (Amendment) Act 2003.

Suicide Act 1961.

Theft Act 1968, sections 1 and 15.

Theft Act 1978.

Theft (Amendment) Act 1996.

White Paper Protection of Vulnerable Adults (POVA) 2000.

Who Decides, 1997.

Williams K. *The Oxford handbook of criminology*, 7th ed. Oxford: Oxford University Press, 2012.

Equality, diversity and inclusivity

Chapter outline

Introduction

From a bioethical perspective, every person deserves to be treated fairly. The principles of justice and beneficence, and non-maleficence and autonomy also apply. The central notion is that service users should be afforded fair treatment, not 'the same' or 'equally'; the care delivered should be patient-centred and based on individual needs (NHS Constitution, 2015). Equality means that individuals should have access to a fair distribution of resources, without discrimination.

The concept of human rights and equality originates from the end of the Second World War, from which an international treaty emerged:

> All human beings are born free and equal in dignity and rights. They are endowed with reason and conscience and should act towards one another in a spirit of brotherhood,
>
> (United Nations, 1948b)

Under the auspices of the United Nations, the Universal Declaration of Human Rights 1948 came into being, recognizing, that, *inter alia*:

Article 2: Everyone is entitled to all the rights and freedoms set forth in this Declaration, without distinction of any kind, such as race, colour, sex, language, religion, political or other opinion, national or social origin, property, birth or other status.

This is applicable to health care, and if the NMC Code (2018); the law; and, by implication, ethical principles are followed, this means that the nurse must balance patients' interests according to their needs as well as subject to available resources.

Diversity includes recognition of individual differences and is defined as
1. the condition of having or being composed of differing elements: variety; especially the inclusion of different types of people (as people of different races or cultures) in a group or organization <programs intended to promote diversity in schools>.
2. an instance of being composed of differing elements or qualities: an instance of being diverse <a diversity of opinion>

(Merriam Dictionary)

What is discrimination-the legal basis?

The concept of 'discrimination' is not easy to define, especially as it is widely used within a variety of differing contexts. The law recognizes the subjective element which the victim needs to demonstrate when they bring their case to court – that they were treated differently. The onus is on a defendant to prove that they did treat the complainant fairly.

There are four main types of discrimination.

Direct discrimination
This means treating one person worse than another person because of a protected characteristic. For example, a promotion comes up at work. The employer believes that people's memories get worse as they get older so doesn't tell one of his older employees about it, because he thinks the employee wouldn't be able to do the job.

Indirect discrimination
This can happen when an organisation puts a rule or a policy or a way of doing things in place which has a worse impact on someone with a protected characteristic than someone without one. For example, a local authority is planning to redevelop some of its housing. It decides to hold consultation events in the evening. Many of the female residents complain that they cannot attend these meetings because of childcare responsibilities.

Harassment
This means people cannot treat you in a way that violates your dignity, or creates a hostile, degrading, humiliating or offensive environment. For example, a man with Down's syndrome is visiting a pub with friends. The bar staff make derogatory and offensive comments about him, which upset and offend him.

Victimisation
This means people cannot treat you unfairly if you are taking action under the Equality Act (like making a complaint of discrimination), or if you are supporting someone else who is doing so. For example, an employee makes a complaint of sexual harassment at work and is dismissed as a consequence.

(Human Rights Commission)

Indirect discrimination appears to be the most challenging one as it is not always evident if a condition or practice is in place, with the effect that individuals who may happen to fall under one of the nine protected characteristics, such as, gender, sex, maternity, race or religion (Equality Act 2010), are disadvantaged. This is commonly found in employment law; for example, it may relate to headwear or clothes.

Box 8.1 Thinking point

1   A fertility clinic refuses to offer services to a woman who happens to be in a same-sex relationship. This constitutes direct discrimination on grounds of sexual orientation.
2   The police stop a group of six rowdy multi-racial youths who were 'messing about' down the High Street. They arrest the only black youth in the group, letting the others go with a warning, claiming that that he was the only one they saw throwing object (though this is disputed by bystanders) This constitutes direct discrimination on grounds of race.

Box 8.2 Case: Webb v EMO Air Cargo (UK) Ltd (14 July 1994) EOR57A

The European Court of Justice rules that it is contrary to the Equal Treatment Directive to dismiss a woman employed for an unlimited term who, shortly after her recruitment, is found to be pregnant, notwithstanding that she was recruited initially to replace another employee during the latter's maternity leave and even though the employer would have dismissed a male employee engaged for this purpose who required a leave of absence at the relevant time for medical or other reasons.

https://www.xperthr.co.uk/law-reports/sick-man-defence-barred/63570/?c-mpid=ILC|PROF|HRPIO-2013-110-XHR_free_content_links|ptod_article&s-fid=701w0000000uNMa

---

It is clear that the Code of Professional Conduct and Ethics (NMC, 2018) requires of nurses the provision of non-discriminatory care for all service users.

Everyone counts. We maximize our resources for the benefit of the whole community and make sure nobody is excluded, discriminated against or left behind. It is clear that some people need more help, and that difficult decisions may need to be taken within the context of scarce or limited resources. The challenge for healthcare professionals is to ensure a fair distribution.

A patient's treatment should be dependent on their individual needs and on the basis of prioritizing on what those needs may be. To those receiving care, certain practices may be interpreted as discriminatory. A patient's needs are those which contribute to their good health: as stated, 'The enjoyment of the highest attainable standard of health is one of the fundamental rights of every human being without distinction of race, religion, political belief, economic or social condition' (WHO Constitution, 1946).

Furthermore, according to the NHS Constitution (2015a) (Para 3a, 2015), a service user has a right '... not to be unlawfully discriminated against in the provision of NHS services including on grounds of gender, race, disability, age, sexual orientation, religion, belief, gender reassignment, pregnancy and maternity or marital or civil part-nership status'.

Disability is an important area linked with court cases related to service provision and employment law. A number of anti-discrimination case laws considered reasonable adjustment in healthcare provision.

Box 8.3 Case: Paulley v First Group plc 2017UKSC 4

The Commission funded Mr Paulley in his case against First Group. Mr Paulley, a wheel-chair user, was prevented from boarding a bus because a child in a buggy was in the disabled space. The Supreme Court found that bus companies must do more to cater to the needs of wheelchair users. This means that the driver should take further steps to pressure a non-wheelchair user into making space for wheelchair users rather than just accepting that a non-wheelchair user cannot move. Bus companies should have clear policies in place and give training to drivers to help them to remove any barriers which wheelchair users face.

https://www.equalityhumanrights.com/en/legal-casework/legal-cases

---

Anti-discriminatory practice was also required in service provision and by employment law, for example, the Race Relations Act 1976 or the Disability Discrimination Act 1995 (both now repealed except in the case of the latter, in Northern Ireland).

Box 8.4 Case: Pimlico Plumbers Ltd & Anor v Smith [2018] UKSC 29

Mr Smith worked for Pimlico Plumbers Ltd as a plumber from August 2005 until April 2011. He did not carry out work for anyone else during this period.

He had a heart attack in 2010 and required adjustments to his work. These were not made. He brought a complaint of disability discrimination.

Pimlico Plumbers argued that the arrangement was a business-to-business relationship. If correct, Mr Smith would have been without protection of the Equality Act 2010.

The Supreme Court found that Mr Smith's employment situation fell within the defini-tion of 'employment' in the Equality Act and so he should be protected by equality law.

https://www.equalityhumanrights.com/en/legal-casework/legal-cases

---

Another common example in healthcare provision is discrimination against older people. It is also clear that while some patients are aware of and are able to assert their right not to be discriminated against, many may not be prepared to complain or may simply lack the knowledge and ability to do so. Where discrimination is established there may not only be breach of an ethical principle but also legal consequences and/or implications for professional registration. Discrimination goes to the heart of patients' fundamental human rights, which must be respected as 'all men and women are created equal and independent … they derive rights inherent and inalienable, among which are the preservation of life and liberty and the pursuit of happiness' (Jefferson, 1950, p. 423).

All types of discrimination involve a breach of fundamental human rights through mistreatment or treatment of one person less favourably in comparison to another, as well as the positive aspect where the favoured individual is given privileged or preferential treatment, again, in comparison to others. This is unacceptable in nursing as the result is unfairness and unequal provision of care. This is the reason why discrimination should be tackled as an infringement of patients' rights as much as that of any other citizen in a democratic society.

The negative aspect, that one or more patients is given preferential treatment, should also be considered, even if this means that this may be difficult to prove. The effect on the disadvantaged person(s) is the same, if they were treated less favourably and made to feel excluded. Alleged victim(s) may therefore have grounds for discrimination under the law. This is clearly in breach of ethical principles (which are embraced by the Beauchamp and Childress' Bioethical, Principlism framework (2013). This means that patients in their care should be treated fairly and neither as 'favourites' nor as 'outcasts'. This is also reflected in the Code of Professional Conduct and Ethics (NMC, 2018).

Prejudice is associated with discrimination and has been defined as 'hostile or negative attitudes based on ignorance and faulty or incomplete knowledge. It is characterized by a tendency to assign identical characteristics to whole groups regardless of individual variations' (Twitchin and Demuth, 1985, p. 170). It is possible for individual prejudices to influence treatment decisions; however, nurses should rise above this in order to demonstrate their respect for ethical principle of justice or fairness as well as refraining from discriminatory treatment based on any deeply rooted, stereotyped attitudes which may be prejudicial towards individuals or a certain group of people.

Box 8.5 Thinking point

Ms C is a 60-year-old a retired Buddhist schoolteacher who is a revolving-door patient with multiple admissions via A&E. She has also a history of complaints and threats of litigation with the aim of getting her own way. She is admitted into accidents and emergency for investigations for abdominal pain and nausea. As a result, she appears to be given preferential treatment in comparison to other patients. On this occasion, she is not happy that the on-call surgeons are in theatre, carrying out an emergency road traffic accident operation. She has settled since coming in but now demands immediate attention. You also have other patients with their own needs.

How is care prioritized for a number of users, for example young, old, disabled, and different genders and religions, with different needs?

What does the nursing and midwifery Council (NMC) require of you in prioritizing needs for this vis-à-vis those of other patients?

Emergence of anti-discrimination legislation, the Equality Act 2010

The Disability Discrimination Act 1995. The aim of the Equality Act 2010 is to provide protection from discrimination for any members of the society-at-large. Prior to this anti-discrimination was piecemeal and the Equality Act brought anti-discrimination legislation based on the following key ones; Sex Discrimination Act 1975, Race Relations Act 1976 and Disability Discrimination Act 1995.

The Equality Act (EA) 2010 legally protects people from discrimination not only in the workplace but also in wider society. This replaces nine pieces of legislation by updating and harmonizing the law on equality and diversity, and it also reinforces what is ethically right as it outlaws discrimination (Article 14, Human Rights Act 1998, European Convention on Human Rights 1950). The EA 2010 has two main purposes:

1. To harmonize all discrimination law, and to strengthen the law to support progress on equality.
2. To bring together and redefine previous legislation and bring this under one umbrella. Most of the existing legislation has been or updated.

This brings all pieces of discrimination legislation under the same umbrella. The statute redefines the grounds for discrimination. Owing to the potential difficulty in providing evidence, or proving that discrimination may have taken place, it is no wonder that victims may be reluctant to come forward. This means that the extent may never be known. Some victims do not have faith in the system or in justice and hence may choose not to report discrimination.

It replaced and harmonizes previous anti-discrimination law, making the law easier to understand and strengthening protection in some situations. It sets out the different ways in which it's unlawful to treat someone. However reprehensible the concept of discrimination per se may sound, there is, in fact, no automatic recognition of it by the law; the law recognizes discrimination as it is only within certain defined parameters. It could be argued that ethical or moral principles would dictate otherwise. Through legislation, Parliament has redefined grounds for discrimination recognizing a diverse society. Grounds for discrimination – the protected characteristics which are grounds for complaint in law – these include:

- age,
- disability,
- gender reassignment,
- marriage and civil partnership,
- pregnancy and maternity,
- race,
- religion or belief,
- sex, and
- sexual orientation.

(Section 4, Human Rights Act 2010)

The Equality Act 2010 now applies to England, Wales and Scotland but not to Northern Ireland. This legislation is an attempt to consider all forms of discrimination under the same umbrella. In reality, it is more probably based on anecdotal evidence only that some types of discrimination will be more common than others. The Equality Commission's main aim is promoting and 'encouraging', with limited powers of enforcement, and is perhaps one of the weaknesses of the law in the area of discrimination. The aim is to create 'fairness' (Government Equalities Office, 2013). Since October 2013, it has been unlawful to victimize anyone who has made a complaint on discrimination.

The precursor of the EA 2010 was Equality Act (EA) 2006 (which is now obsolete), which was to a point effective but not up-to-date with modern-day trends as it targeted discrimination as an umbrella. It also aimed to be a legal 'umbrella', which attempted to bring together all types of discrimination. Most of the existing anti-discrimination legislation remains intact, Monaghan (2013) and this statute aims to integrate and coordinate the fight against discrimination by having one central body, the commission. The importance of this area of legislation is that victims should feel that they have access to justice and are not put off by any red tape. The effectiveness of anti-discrimination legislation depends on the willingness of victims to complain. The difficulty is that while some persons on the receiving end may not wish to complain about discrimination, others who lack the competence, such as incapacitated patients or those who lack knowledge about their rights, may do nothing. Some patients may feel that they do not wish to 'rock the boat' and, indeed, choose to put up with discrimination in the case of victimization.

Owing to their physical and possible mental incapacity, a large number of patients may fall into this category, often being impaired (from a physical or mental incapacity) or having limited ability to function. This is an important area of law which the nurse needs to understand as they provide care for this group of (disabled) patients. It is the impairment of any part or parts of the body on which disability focusses and the absence of or limitation of 'bodily mechanism' (Oliver, in Helman, 2007). This is seen by some as the basis for determining the presence of disability.

Disability discrimination

Reasonable adjustment is necessary for providing fairness (including access), where resources are limited, or standard arrangements and service may be inadequate. This happens when services provision does not meet the needs of those individuals included under the nine protected characteristics. This is defined by statute, and the duty to make reasonable adjustments (defined below,)

> (1) Where this Act imposes a duty to make reasonable adjustments on a person, this section, sections 21 and 22 and the applicable Schedule apply; and for those purposes, a person on whom the duty is imposed is referred to as A.
> (2) The duty comprises the following three requirements.
> (3) The first requirement is a requirement, where a provision, criterion or practice of A's puts a disabled person at a substantial disadvantage in relation to a relevant matter in comparison with persons who are not disabled, to take such steps as it is reasonable to have to take to avoid the disadvantage.
> (4) The second requirement is a requirement, where a physical feature puts a disabled person at a substantial disadvantage in relation to a relevant matter in comparison with persons who are not disabled, to take such steps as it is reasonable to have to take to avoid the disadvantage.
> (5) The third requirement is a requirement, where a disabled person would, but for the provision of an auxiliary aid, be put at a substantial disadvantage in relation to a relevant matter in comparison with persons who are not disabled, to take such steps as it is reasonable to have to take to provide the auxiliary aid
>
> (Equality Act 2010, Section 20)

For government agencies, such as Social Services and the Department of Employment, any persons who are disabled were covered by the Disabled Persons (Employment) Act 1944, Section 1 classification of those with the following:

(1) These include injury, disease or congenital deformity is substantially handicapped in obtaining or keeping employment, or in undertaking work on his own account, of a kind which would be suited to his age, experience and qualifications.

The Disability Discrimination Act (DDA) 1995, Section 20(1), suggested that discrimination exists when there is 'less favourable treatment' of a person with disability. The Equality Act 2010 is a consolidation of and repealed the DDA 1995 (except for Northern Ireland), and focusses on areas such as public transport and housing provision by regulating public authorities to ensure they treat all users fairly. Disability also includes mental illness under the Mental Health Act 1983, Section 1, which includes the following four categories:

1. mental illness,
2. mental impairment,
3. severe mental impairment,
4. psychopathic disorder.

The Human Rights Act 1998 (enacted the European Convention on Human Rights 1950 in the UK) came into force in 2000. It was felt, however, that the issue of discrimination was fragmented, and this culminated in a major change with the enactment of the Equality Act 2010. The catalyst for change was the House of Commons itself in a body which would police the implementation on human rights and related anti-discriminatory legislation; 'an independent commission would be the most effective way of achieving the shared aim of bringing about a culture of respect for human rights' (Joint Committee on Human Rights, 2002–03). Furthermore, it is important to note the differences between the two statutes, the Disability Discrimination Act (DDA) 1995 and the Equality Act (EA) 2010. The EA generally carries forward the protection provided for disabled people by the DDA. However, there are key differences:

- The DDA provided protection for disabled people from direct discrimination only in employment and related areas. The EA protects disabled people against direct discrimination in areas beyond the employment field (such as the supply of goods, facilities and services).
- The EA introduced improved protection from discrimination that occurs because of something connected with a person's disability. This form of discrimination can be justified if it can be shown to be a proportionate means of achieving a legitimate aim.
- The EA introduced the principle of indirect discrimination for disability. Indirect discrimination occurs when something applies in the same way to everybody but has an effect which particularly disadvantages, for example, disabled people. Indirect discrimination may be justified if it can be shown to be a proportionate means of achieving a legitimate aim.
- The EA applies one trigger point ... a duty to make reasonable adjustments for disabled people. This trigger point is where a disabled person would be at a substantial disadvantage compared to non-disabled people if the adjustment was not made.

(Office for Disability Issues [ODI], 2013)

In addition, there are further differences which make it easier for clients with disability to raise a complaint, where discrimination may be subtle, difficult to prove or result from making a complaint, as follows:

- The EA extends protection from harassment that is related to disability. Previously, explicit protection only applied in relation to work. The EA applies this protection to areas beyond work.
- The EA provides protection from direct disability discrimination and harassment where this is based on a person's association with a disabled person, or on a false perception that the person is disabled.
- The EA contains a provision which limits the type of enquiries that a recruiting employer can make about disability and health when recruiting new staff. This provision will help prevent disabled candidates from being unfairly screened out at an early stage of the recruitment process.

(Office for Disability Issues [ODI], 2013)

Box 8.6 Thinking point: age and sexual orientation discrimination

A, a gay man, aged 70, is a retired ballet dancer. He emigrated to the UK from the United States with B, his now ex-partner, and has been living in the UK for the last ten years. He is admitted after suffering a nervous breakdown following the end of his relationship. He is admitted to a busy orthopaedic ward for leg surgery following a road traffic accident, causing a fractured femur. His operation goes well, though his rehabilitation is progressing slowly. The ward nurses put him in a side room due to complaints from another patient.

He is partially sighted and registered blind, which makes him increasingly dependent on others for some activities of living. As he is in a side room, he tends to be left until last for washing and dressing. He is now suffering from depression after splitting up with B, his partner of ten years (an older man, 20 years his senior), who has recently left him for another man.

Consider the issues which you think may amount to discrimination.

1   A complains that he heard a staff member making homophobic comments.
2   He says he feels isolated and that 'no one cares'.
3   How would you ensure that you empower the patient?
4   Now apply the NMC Code (2018) to discrimination.

Age discrimination

The National Service Framework (NSF) for Older People 2001 recognizes that elderly people may be discriminated against and sets a benchmark for healthcare professionals to aspire towards when delivering care for elderly people. This is a requirement for Standard 1 (rooting out age discrimination).

NHS services should be provided, regardless of age, on the basis of clinical needs alone. Social care services will not use age in their eligibility criteria or policies, to restrict access to available services. The aim of NSFs such as the above is to improve national standards and hence the quality of care for patients. Breach of such standards does not mean an automatic breach of statutory provisions. However, where a service provider fails to meet these standards, this may be evidence of liability in law, as when they fail in their duty of care to the patient in areas such as tort law. An example of an important aspect of discrimination which may affect the elderly in the provision of care is the provision of care packages. It is possible that this may be seen as a soft target in the need to save money, and effectively discriminates against the elderly DoH 2001, 2012). This is more evident in Mental Health, Royal College of Psychiatry (2018) Suffering in silence: age inequality in older people's mental health care. Discrimination takes place as a result of providers having stigma and prejudice. Prejudice has been defined above. The nurse responsible for the care of an older person should never make assumptions, based on physical appearance and impairments alone, that the patient lacks mental capacity and will therefore be unaware of discrimination.

Racial discrimination

In most instances the concept of 'discrimination' takes many forms, with a range of definitions. The difficulty of racial discrimination is that it depends on a subjective perception or interpretation of concerning the victim of the alleged racist act.

A person discriminates against another in any circumstances relevant for the purposes of any provision of this act if

- on racial grounds he treats that other less favourably than he treats or would treat other persons; or
- he applies to that other a requirement or condition which he applies or would apply equally to persons not of the same racial group as that other.

(Section 1 of Race Relations Act 1976
[now repealed by the Equality Act 2010])

Again, the onus or burden of proof is on the defendant to show that there was no unfair treatment on grounds of race. When patients lack either mental or physical capacity, it may be very difficult to establish discrimination on the grounds of race. Discrimination on the grounds of race may also result from indirect discrimination by way of victimization. A study by Shah and Priestley (2001) showed that subjects who came from black and ethnic minority backgrounds had experienced discriminatory practices while receiving care. They perceived this to be based on their race when they compared their treatment with that of others.

Gender reassignment

The government has acknowledged that the Gender Recognition (GRA) Act 2004, which aimed to allow trans people to change their gender, needs reform, hence the launch of a consultation in July 2018. Gender dysphoria is a medical diagnosis.

A diagnosis of gender dysphoria can usually be made after an in-depth assessment carried out by two or more specialists.

This may require several sessions, carried out a few months apart, and may involve discussions with people you are close to, such as members of your family or your partner.

The assessment will determine if you have gender dysphoria and what their needs are, which could include:

- whether there's a clear mismatch between your biological sex and gender identity
- whether you have a strong desire to change your physical characteristics as a result of any mismatch
- how you're coping with any difficulties of a possible mismatch
- how your feelings and behaviours have developed over time
- what support you have, such as friends and family
- The assessment may also involve a more general assessment of your physical and psychological health.

(NHS UK, 2019)

A limited number of people have changed their gender,

Since the GRA 2004, came into force, only 4,910 people have legally changed their gender. This is fewer than the number of trans respondents to the government's LGBT survey, who were clear that they wanted legal recognition but had not applied because they found the current process too bureaucratic, expensive and intrusive.

(GOV.UK, 2018)

Classification of discrimination, objective justification

Can discrimination ever be justified? There are exceptions in law where 'objective' discrimination may be legitimate:

- the health, safety and welfare of individuals
- running an efficient service
- requirements of a business
- desire to make profit.

Example
A hospital advertises a surgeon's job for which it requires at least ten years' experience. You can't meet this requirement because you've taken time off work to care for your children. As you're a woman, this looks like indirect discrimination because of sex. But the hospital may be able to justify this, if it can show that the job can't be done properly without that amount of experience. This is likely to be a legitimate aim.

(Citizen Advice UK)

It is difficult to establish how widespread other types of discrimination are in health care as people may not raise concerns. Vulnerable people may be unwilling or unable to make a complaint under legislation such as the articles in Schedule 1 of the Human Rights Act 1998, European Convention on Human Rights 1950. This included discrimination on grounds such as gender, sexual orientation and religious beliefs. Discrimination on grounds of gender is now forbidden in the Equality Act 2010, while discrimination on the grounds of sexual orientation is outlawed; the passing of the Civil Partnership Act 2004 afforded same-sex couples the right to civil unions with the latest legislation, the Marriage (Same Sex Couples) Act 2013 (c. 30), now affording same-sex couples the same rights as heterosexual couples. Furthermore, discrimination on religion or on religious belief is now also outlawed under the Employment Equality (Religion or Belief) Regulations 2003.

The law (under the Equality Act 2010) now recognizes all the above aspects and contexts of discrimination. It is hoped that nurses can now turn to their own ethics, their professional code of conduct, national benchmarks such as the NSF for Older People 2001 and their local policies and guidelines which should all enshrine equal rights to fair treatment and care for all patients.

Box 8.7 Thinking point

Jane is a junior qualified staff nurse who has worked on an acute care of the elderly ward for six months post-qualifying. One patient, Mrs S (a widow, aged 77, who is a religious woman from West Africa) happens to live on the same street as Jane. She speaks limited English and does not communicate much with other staff members as she says they do not like people of her colour. She likes Jane, whom she calls 'a daughter'; her colleagues are concerned about boundaries.

However, it has also become clear that Jane knows the patient from links with her church. Jane spends time talking to Mrs S in her own language, to the exclusion of other patients and staff. Jane's response is that the patient is lonely and needs some advocacy.

1   Find out about your organization's anti-discrimination policies.
2   Based on this information, what advice would you give to Mrs S and Jane?

Diversity and Inclusivity

Diversity means;

> the fact of many different types of things or people being included in something; a range of different things or people
>
> Cambridge Dictionary

Diversity includes a range of people from different backgrounds, based on the nine protected characteristics in the Equality Act 2010. Diversity is about recognising people's differences and these should be seen as strengths and not weaknesses.

Through avoiding stereotyping and engaging inclusivity and recognition of the fact that people are different we should not take who we see at face value, not based on the surface (Kreps and Kunimoto [1994] Iceberg model). Inclusivity means that there may be aspects of a person that we do not see 'deep-down'. At best this may apply to disability, age, sex, gender or sexuality, though it is applicable to the nine characteristics of the EA 2010. Inclusivity also means respecting and facilitating the service users' preferred customs, from a simple issue such as what they would like to be called to advance statements which may be based on their customs and religion. The latter should be respected, though they are not legally binding. Advanced decision, on the other hand, is binding in its entirety. The patient's wishes may be in a written format or confirmed through communicating with the patient and their loved ones. This ranges from dietary preferences and last offices.

Some progress has been made so far under the EA 2010. One area in which progress has been made is disability, the definition of which has been broadened to include clients with long-term conditions:

A person has a disability if –

(a) P has a physical or mental impairment, and
(b) the impairment has a substantial and long-term adverse effect on their ability to carry out normal day-to-day activities.

The recent consultation may have a proposed statute, which is a Gender Recognition Act 2004 which will provide for self-determination of gender for people who undergo a procedure to change their sex rather than a medical diagnosis of gender dysphoria. It is by being more proactive and engaging in promoting equality and diversity that we tackle discrimination. Healthcare staff need to be aware that even the well-meaning individuals may have unconscious bias against some people who fall within the nine protected characteristics. Recent changes extend the law on forming civil partnership to the law now allowing persons who are not of the same sex to have a civil partnership (Civil Partnerships, Marriages and Deaths (Registration etc) Act 2019). This was preceded by the following case: *(R on the application of Steinfeld and Keidan) (Appellants) v Secretary of State for International Development (in substitution for the Home Secretary and the Education Secretary) (Respondent) [2018] UKSC 32.* This case was brought to the Supreme Court by a mixed-sex couple on the grounds of breach of their human rights.

Conclusion

Unfair or unequal treatment of patients may be discriminatory. The Equalities Commission has as its main objective the promotion of equality and diversity in all aspects of life (EA 2006, above). The problem with discrimination is that under present UK law, the alleged victim has to make a claim about what they may perceive as discrimination. This may not pose any difficulty for patients who have the mental capacity. For those who lack capacity, however, they may be unaware of any discriminatory acts affecting their care, hence the importance of the Mental Capacity Act 2005 to safeguard their interests.

On the issue of equality and diversity, nurses and healthcare professionals should recognize that there are differences among people who are their patients. Their patients are entitled to non-discriminatory treatment under human rights legislation and in ethics. While some differences may be visible, others may not be visible or obvious. This means that making assumptions about a patient's capacity (physical or mental) or their needs can never be justified, as this may result in discrimination. The standard of care that nurses deliver should be influenced not purely by the law and by their own ethical beliefs but also by a professional culture, which recognizes and values patients as individuals. They should always respect the patient's human rights. Together, the

EA 2006, the Race Relations (Amendment) Act 2000, the Disability Discrimination Act 2005 and related statutes have aimed to make it easier for healthcare providers and others such as social services to have an integrated approach to the fair treatment of users in the elimination of discrimination.

Anti-discriminatory practice is key to 'fairness' in ethics (Beauchamp and Childress, 2013) and in nursing. A nurse responsible for providing care must respond to the needs of patients from 'diverse' backgrounds. They need to avoid favouritism or disadvantaging any individual patients and care for all their patients without fear and favour. Providing preferential treatment for one patient happens to detract from other patients' rights while also compromising the treatment of other 'less advantaged' patients. This may mean that the care given to all patients falls below the expected standards of a person possessing their skills under the Bolam principle (see in Chapter 2). All professional codes of conduct for healthcare personnel require from their members fair treatment as well as non-discrimination of patients or clients.

Some improvement in the focus of the aim of legislation in improving equality and diversity is evident since the passing of the Equality Act 2010, which attempts to bring grounds for discrimination under an 'umbrella'. In practice, it may not be as easy for an alleged victim to prove this or to be courageous to bring a complaint forward without fear of victimization. There may still be grounds of discrimination which may still not be directly recognized by and enforceable under existing law. One example is discrimination on the grounds of social status or class. The fact is that discrimination may often be subtle and difficult to prove.

References

Beauchamp T and Childress J. *Bioethics*, 8th ed. Oxford: Oxford University Press, 2013.

Cambridge Dictionary. Available online at: https://dictionary.cambridge.org/dictionary/english/diversity (accessed on 20th April 2020).

Citizen Advice UK. Available online at: https://www.citizensadvice.org.uk/law-and-courts/discrimination/what-are-the-different-types-of-discrimination/justifying-discrimination/ (accessed on 12th August 2019).

Civil Partnership Act 2004.

Civil Partnerships, Marriages and Deaths (Registration etc) Act 2019.

Department of Health (2001) National service framework for older people. Available online at: https://www.gov.uk/government/publications/quality-standards-for-care-services-for-older-people (accessed on 18th July 2019).

Department of Health (2012) Implementing a ban on age discrimination in the NHS – making effective, appropriate decisions. Available online at: https://www.gov.uk/government/publications/implementing-a-ban-on-age-discrimination-in-the-nhs-making-effective-appropriate-decisions (accessed on 3rd July 2019).

Disability Discrimination Act 1995.

Disability Discrimination Act (DDA) 1995, Section 20(1).

Disabled Persons (Employment) Act 1944.

Employment Equality (Religion or Belief) Regulations 2003.

Equality Act 2010.

Equality Act 2010, Section 20.

Equality Commission. Available online at: https://www.equalityhumanrights.com/en/advice-and-guidance/your-rights-under-equality-act-2010 (accessed on 2nd August 2019).

Equality Commission. Available online at: https://www.equalityhumanrights.com/en (accessed on 11th December 2019).

European Convention on Human Rights 1950.

Gender Recognition (GRA) Act 2004.

GOV.UK (2018) Reform of the Gender Recognition Act 2004. Available online at: https://www.gov.uk/government/consultations/reform-of-the-gender-recognition-act-2004 (accessed on 24th October 2019).

Human Rights Act 1998.

Human Rights Commission. Available online at: https://www.equalityhumanrights.com/en/advice-and guidance/your-rights-under-equality-act-2010 (accessed on 19th October 2019).

Jefferson T. Rough draft of the American declaration of independence. In Boyd J, ed., *Papers of Thomas Jefferson*. Princeton: Princeton University Press, p. 423, 1950.

Kreps GL and Kunimoto EN. Effective communication in multicultural health care. London: Jessica Kingsley, 1994.

Marriage (Same Sex Couples) Act 2013 (c. 30).

Mental Health Act 1983, Section 1.

Merriam Dictionary. Available online at: https://www.merriam-webster.com/dictionary/diversity (accessed on 23rd December 2019).

Monaghan K. *Monaghan on equality law*, 2nd ed. Oxford: Oxford University Press, 2013.

National Service Framework (NSF) for Older People 2001.

NHS Constitution, NHS choices (2015) A para 3a. Available online at: https://www.gov.uk/government/publications/the-nhs-constitution-for-england (accessed on 18th October 2019).

NHS UK (2019) Available online at: https://www.nhs.uk/conditions/gender-dysphoria/ (accessed on 11th December 2019).

Nursing and Midwifery Council. *Code of professional conduct and ethics*. London: NMC, 2018.

Office for Disability Issues (ODI) (2013) Available online at: https://www.gov.uk/government/organisations/office-for-disability-issues (accessed on 20th August 2019).

Oliver M. In Helman C, ed., *Culture, health and illness*, 5th ed. London: Hodder Arnold, 2007.

Paulley v First Group plc 2017UKSC 4.

Pimlico Plumbers Ltd & Anor v Smith [2018] UKSC 29.

R. (on the application of Steinfeld and Keidan) (Appellants) v Secretary of State for International Development (in substitution for the Home Secretary and the Education Secretary) (Respondent) [2018] UKSC 32.

Race Relations Act 1976.

Shah S, Priestley M. Better services, better health: the healthcare experiences of black and minority ethnic disabled people. 2001. Available online at: https://disability-studies.leeds.ac.uk/wp-content/uploads/sites/40/2011/10/LIPfinalreport.pdf (accessed on 20th June 2019).

Twitchin J and Demuth C. *Multi-cultural education: Views from the classroom*, 2nd ed. London: BBC, 1985.

United Nations (1948) The universal declaration of human rights. Available online at: https://www.un.org/en/universal-declaration-human-rights/ (accessed on 20th July 2018).

WHO Constitution (1946) WHO remains firmly committed to the principles set out in the preamble to the constitution. Available online at: https://www.who.int/about/who-we-are/constitution (accessed on 2nd October 2019).

9 End-of-life care, decision-making

Chapter outline

Introduction

This chapter explores one of the most important aspects of life and care for people towards their final continuum of life. Based on everyday experience, human mortality is a certain and indisputable fact. It is not a question of whether this occurs; rather it is a question of when it occurs. Dying has been described as 'a human process in the same way that being born is a normal and all-human process' (Kubler-Ross, 1991, p. 10). Nowadays, it is much more difficult to determine when death occurs due to advanced medical science interventions (Campbell et al., 2005). The core ethical question on the end of life issue is how and when the end of life should be facilitated.

There are different views at both ends of the spectrum – on the one hand, absolute preservation of life (and delaying the inevitable), and on the other hand, allowing death or 'letting go', if not assisting or hastening the end. In either case, there is a potential conflict of interests, between the patient's best interests and those of other stakeholders and possibly those of society as a whole, in consideration of the ethical and legal implications. Society's motives may be driven by caring and altruistic concerns to prolong life, or (cynically) economic reasons may play a part, by considering the costs of maintaining what seems to be a futile life. The court's role is usually a balancing act and may find that there is no absolute obligation on doctors to prolong life regardless if treatment outcomes are poor.

Under certain provisions, states assume their right through legislation to determine when a life can be ended, actively or passively. This may be in the case of retributive justice, when a capital sentence is allowed for murder, on the basis of the 'life-for-life' principle. Sometimes it could be argued in ethics and law that justifiable homicide (one person killing another) will be accepted, but this is only in clearly defined circumstances, such as in self-defence or as an act of war.

End of life and euthanasia

In medical terms, death is defined as

> the cessation of all vital functions of the body including the heartbeat, brain activity (including the brain stem), and breathing.
>
> (Medical Dictionary)

This may be described as 'end of life' for an infant or adult, occurring at a later stage of life, usually at the end of the spectrum, unlike abortion, which is termination of life following conception and living. Some ancient Greek moral philosophers believed that there might be situations in which euthanasia would be justifiable provided that it was 'easy and gentle'. The word 'euthanasia' had a somewhat wider connotation then, having no specific reference to so-called 'mercy killing' (Teichman, 1996, p. 65). In consideration of patient care by physicians, the Hippocratic Oath (500 BC) required physicians to sustain and enhance the quality of life of their patients. These are related to a general consensus evident in professional codes of conduct across disciplines of healthcare professionals including nursing. This means that most ethical philosophies and religions view life as a gift from a supernatural 'being', some form of deity or 'Mother Nature'. This entity is seen as having the ultimate right to give or to take life. There, however, appears to be no consensus on the stage at which life begins and equally no agreement as to when life should end. Medical science can now sustain life at a basic level to a greater extent than it could in the time of the ancient Greeks. Incidentally, the legal definition of death is much broader, to include biological life, while the clinical-medical one is limited to brain stem dysfunction as the basis for determining death, a persistent vegetative state (PVS). The law on human rights considers the fact that every patient is entitled to a right to life (Article 2 of European Convention on Human Rights (1950), (Human Rights Act 1998); hence, this has been used as a basis for litigation to assert that right.

Everyone's right to life shall be protected by the law. No one shall be deprived of their life intentionally, save in the execution of a sentence of a court following their conviction of a crime for which this penalty is provided by the law.

Article 2 of Human Rights Act 1998

This, nevertheless, should be qualified. There are many definitions of euthanasia, and the preferred one serves as a starting point for defining euthanasia as death:

> (death) the cessation of life; permanent cessation of all vital bodily functions. For legal and medical purposes, the following definition of death has been proposed-the irreversible cessation of all of the following: (1) total cerebral function, usually assessed by EEG as flat-line (2) spontaneous function of the respiratory system, and (3) spontaneous function of the circulatory system...
>
> brain d[eath]. irreversible brain damage as manifested by absolute unresponsiveness to all stimuli, absence of all spontaneous muscle activity, including respiration, shivering, etc., and an isoelectric electroencephalogram for 30 minutes, all

in the absence of hypothermia or intoxication by central nervous system depressants. Called also irreversible coma and cerebral d[eath].

(Dorland's Illustrated Medical Dictionary)

Death is difficult to establish; 'as a result of developments in modern medical technology, doctors no longer associate death exclusively with breathing and heart-beat, and it has come to be accepted that death occurs when the brain, and in particular the brain stem, has been destroyed' (Lord Goff in the following case).

The definitions of 'life' and 'death' are the subject of debate throughout healthcare professional frameworks. Consider the following definition of end of life below:

Box 9.1 Case: Airedale NHS Trust v Bland [1993] 1 All ER 821

Anthony David bland, a Liverpool football Club fan, then aged 17, attended the Hillsborough ground for a match. During the disastrous course of events of that day, he was crushed and subsequently suffered brain damage from a lack of oxygen supply to his brain, with resulting irreversible brain damage. By the time the case went to court, he had been in a persistent vegetative state (PVS) for some time. The question for the court was whether his artificial feeding should be discontinued, and with the agreement of the consultant and the family, this was allowed.

People are 'approaching the end of life' when they are likely to die within the next 12 months. This includes people whose death is imminent (expected within a few hours or days) and those with

- advanced, progressive, incurable conditions
- general frailty and co-existing conditions that mean they are expected to die within 12 months
- existing conditions if they are at risk of dying from a sudden acute crisis in their condition
- life-threatening acute conditions caused by sudden catastrophic events.

(NICE, 2017)

As applied to the clinical setting, it is a reasonable expectation in civil law and in ethics that healthcare professionals owe a duty of care to provide a reasonable standard of care to maintain the welfare of patients under their care, see *Donoghue v Stevenson [1932], AC 532*; discussed below. The primary goal should be to promote health as well as to save lives. A dilemma may arise when healthcare professionals must engage in end of life decisions. Healthcare professionals may experience contrasting roles, from fighting to save a life to accepting the fact that treatment may be futile with death being inevitable. It has been suggested that 'nurses are expected to implement ethical decisions to withdraw treatment when they have not been party to the decision-making process' (Viney, 1996, p. 182) in the first place. The most important ethical question is to determine whether in their role they can foresee circumstances in which it is justifiable to either actively or passively terminate that life by withdrawing treatment. The patient or their representatives must be involved in decision-making (NHS Constitution, 2015).

The literary origin of the word *Eu-thanasia* is the Greek translation for a 'good-death'. It has been argued by some that the concept of euthanasia should include a positive 'enabling' aspect which includes the patient's autonomy and the right to choose (Davies, 1998).

Healthcare professionals, in general, and doctors, in particular, face a dilemma when trying to establish a patient's capacity to choose treatment which, in their professional judgement, they may consider to be futile. This task is difficult considering that a patient's judgement may be influenced by poor physical and/or psychological impairment resulting from disease. The ability to establish the patient's best interests is even more difficult when they (the patient) are mentally incapacitated or have intermittent consciousness and rationality. The question posed here is whether there are any circumstances where substitution of that judgement by another person's judgement would be justifiable. There follows a definition of 'best interests' with an explanation for determining them.

(1) In determining for the purposes of this Act, what is in a person's best interests, the person making the determination must consider all the circumstances appearing to him to be relevant.
(2) In particular, he must take the following steps.
(3) He must consider (a) whether it is likely that the person will at some time have capacity in relation to the matter in question and, (b) if it appears likely that he will, when that is likely to be.
(4) He must, so far as reasonably practicable, permit and encourage the person to participate, or to improve his ability to participate, as fully as possible in any act done for him and any decision affecting him.

(Mental Capacity Act 2004, section 4)

Active euthanasia

A person may legally take active measures to end their life by consuming a concoction of drugs or by any other means, knowing that that action will end their life, which is suicide. A similar effect may be achieved through the assistance of another person, in which case this becomes 'assisted suicide' as well as the crime of aiding and abetting (Section 2(1) of Suicide Act 1961). These are offences subject to criminal law scrutiny and possible prosecution. Physician-assisted suicide is an alternative to withdrawal of treatment, when a patient requests a doctor to provide them with drugs that will shorten or end life. Euthanasia is murder in the UK. This is on the basis of the following case:

Box 9.2 Case: Regina v Cox [1992] 12 BMLR 38

A 70-year-old woman suffered from advanced stages of arthritis with severe pain. It could not be established how much longer she would have lived but for the administration of a potent substance, resulting in her death. She had suffered from severe arthritis pain for several years, which was not controlled by analgesia. She had requested her consultant, Cox, to put her out of her misery. Dr Cox then knowingly injected her with a lethal dose of potassium chloride resulting in her death. He was initially charged with murder but subsequently found guilty of attempted murder. The judge directing the jury said that 'if it is proved that Dr Cox injected Lillian Boyes with potassium chloride in circumstances which make sure that by that act he intended to kill her, then he is guilty of attempted murder'. The case resulted in a suspended sentence. As the body had been cremated before the case was brought to the attention of the police, it was not proven that the injected potassium was the cause of death.

Physician-assisted suicide may be either voluntary, when a patient is mentally competent and gives permission, or involuntary, when the patient lacks the capacity to make an informed choice, such as in the case of an unconscious patient. Incompetent patients have no legal rights to refuse consent to treatment. There are now new provisions under the Mental Capacity Act 2005, while the Mental Health Act 1983 is replaced by the Mental Health Act 2007, with Adults with Incapacity (Scotland) Act 2000 and Mental Health (Care and Treatment) (Scotland) Act 2003 applicable, respectively. Unless it can be proven otherwise, there is now a presumption in law that every adult patient has the capacity to make an informed decision. The difference between 'suicide' and 'physician-assisted suicide' is that the latter is carried out within a clinical setting and protected by the law in a handful of countries. Physician-assisted euthanasia is illegal under current UK legislation.

Passive euthanasia

This involves those situations in which a patient's treatment is either withdrawn by stopping current treatment or by making a decision that no new interventions will be instituted. One example is where antibiotics may be indicated for treatment of a chest infection and a conscious decision is made not to administer antibiotics because any further treatment would not have any meaningful benefit to the patient. Since *NHS Trust v Bland [1993] 1 All ER 821 HL* (above), in which there is a lack of clarity, it has been the principle that the court's permission must be sought before deciding to withdraw treatment.

Voluntary euthanasia

Voluntary euthanasia involves a patient who possesses the mental capacity to make an informed choice. Such a patient may choose to accept a form of treatment or refuse it even with the awareness that the consequence will be detrimental to their health. A patient's right to exercise autonomy in accepting or refusing treatment should be respected in ethics, since the passing of the Suicide Act 1961, Section 1. In some countries, for example, the Netherlands, voluntary physician-assisted suicide would be granted if the conditions for the relevant framework were satisfied. This is different in the UK, although the Mental Capacity Act 2005 of England and Wales which implements the Convention on the International Protection of Adults (signed at The Hague on 13 January 2000 (cm. 5881)) tips the balance in favour of the patient. On the other hand, doctors and nurses may not be forced to carry out any clinical actions they consider contrary to their professional judgement or which they find morally reprehensible unless this is within the confines of the law. Establishing the 'voluntariness' based on informed consent is at the centre of decision-making.

Involuntary euthanasia

This may apply to situations where a patient lacks the capacity to make a rational choice, and this raises questions on the extent to which, in reality, a patient's autonomy can influence outcomes related to treatment. There has been long-standing provision for a formal proxy to make decisions on behalf of the patient in financial matters (the proxy having been granted a power of attorney) but not regarding treatment. The power of the 'healthcare proxy' was different under Scots law, where the former may, in certain circumstances, make a choice on behalf of the patient. Since the passing of the Mental Capacity Act 2005, however, a deputy in England and Wales and Northern Ireland now has similar powers. This introduces a new dimension and a presumption in law that every adult has the capacity to make an informed decision. An advocate or healthcare proxy with power of attorney may not override a clinical decision. They may only accept or decline.

Adoption of a bioethical framework for decision-making (which is considered as universal in its application) is necessary for healthcare professionals in order to reach the correct decisions related to the end of life. Principlism (or bioethical principles) aims to define basic human rights starting with autonomy, beneficence, non-maleficence and fairness in the decision-making framework, making the four ethical principles an essential part of the medical/nursing ethical framework for decision-making. Beauchamp and Childress (2013) first termed them 'universal'. Euthanasia may be subject to a person's own choice or through 'assistance', whether at the hands of a professional or another person, someone's own actions or the actions of others. An example of own actions is refusal of treatment, which may result in termination of life. The general principle of a patient's right to autonomy was nevertheless altered in the following case:

Box 9.3 Case: Re T (Adult: Refusal of Medical Treatment) [1992] 4 All ER 649, CA

A pregnant woman, aged 20, had suffered serious injuries in a road traffic accident. The injuries included a haemorrhage, which resulted in the birth of a stillborn baby. She had been 34 weeks pregnant and, on admission, had consented to a Caesarean section. Her mother, who was a strict Jehovah's Witness, had then influenced her daughter (Ms T), who subsequently told doctors that she objected to a blood transfusion. Her boyfriend and his father, on the other hand, objected to their decision and sought a judicial review authorizing a blood transfusion as a life-saving measure.

Held: it was held by the Court of appeal (Lord Donaldson's judgement) that

1   Her mental capacity to choose whether to accept a blood transfusion or not had been impaired by her injuries.
2   She had lacked sufficient information to make an informed (rational) decision to accept or refuse treatment.
3   Undue pressure from her mother may have influenced her subsequent decision to appear to reject a blood transfusion.

The courts therefore could not apply the ethical principle of autonomy under these circumstances and ordered a transfusion to be given to Ms T without her consent.

Is Suicide – a Human Right or a Criminal Act?

In consideration of the concept of 'human rights' there is a presumption that every person may make a choice about how and where they lead their lives, and therefore, arguably, this right should include how and when to terminate their own lives. This may be acceptable to some, while others may find this morally reprehensible.

Under Section 1, Suicide Act 1961, suicide is no longer a crime, meaning that prosecution will not follow, but this provision does not necessarily mean that the UK sanctions the act of suicide. Suicide ceased to be a crime, under Section 1, Suicide Act 1961, 'the rule of law whereby it is a crime for a person to commit suicide is hereby abrogated'. However, Section 2(1) of the Suicide Act 1961 states that physician-assisted or 'other person-assisted' suicide is illegal. Other competing interests in society may limit individual rights and choices. A patient's expressed wish to commit suicide may be motivated by unbearable pain and/or depressive illness as well as by social pressures. Assisted suicide takes place when another person is involved, be it a doctor or a layperson.

A person who assists another person to take their life may be charged with murder under Section 1 of the Homicide Act 1957. Furthermore, 'A person who aids, abets, counsels or procures the suicide of another or an attempt by another to commit suicide shall be liable on conviction on indictment to imprisonment for a term not exceeding 14 years', Section 2(1) of Suicide Act 1961, as amended by the Coroners and Justice Act 2009, which provides a definition:

2 Criminal liability for complicity in another's suicide
   (1) A person ('D') commits an offence if –
   (a) D does an act capable of encouraging or assisting the suicide or attempted suicide of another person, and,
   (b) D's act was intended to encourage or assist suicide or an attempt at suicide.

Subject to Section 4 of the Suicide Act 1981, however, where evidence of a suicide pact is present, the charge may be reduced from murder to manslaughter. Section 2(1) of Suicide Act 1961 (above) sets a maximum sentence of 14 years' imprisonment. The above section was unsuccessfully challenged in the case below.

Box 9.4 Case: Pretty v the United Kingdom (European Court of Human Rights), application no. 2346/02, Strasbourg, April 29; [2002]

In this case, a woman with motor neuron disease invoked her right to choose refusal of treatment, under Articles 2, 3 and 8 of the European Convention on the Protection of Human Rights 1950. She sought immunity from prosecution for her husband on assisting her to die with dignity. This was unanimously rejected by the House of Lords, and on appeal, that decision was upheld by the European Court of Human rights.

Mainstream religions such as Christianity, Islam and Judaism do not accept an individual's right to commit suicide on the basis of what is regarded as the 'sanctity of life'. Buddhism also rejects the notion of suicide or self-harm and considers it morally reprehensible and wrong. Some Hindu writers would argue, however, that 'there is a right time (natural) "kala" for death' and also hold that there should be 'the acceptability of willed death, where a man may control his death by refusing to take food or drink' (Morgan and Lawton, 1996, p. 3). They nevertheless believe that only the supernatural or 'Divine Being' has the right to give and take life. Some moral philosophers, such as Kant (1724–1804), propose that under no circumstance should suicide be justifiable. His 'categorical imperative' concept includes a moral duty to do what is right and cannot include suicide as this would be absurd. It is not a question of choice. On the other hand, utilitarianism would argue that whatever course of action produces the greatest benefit or happiness for the greatest number of people should be followed and hence could justify suicide in some circumstances. From a pragmatic point of view, it could be argued that, at least for those with loved ones and dependants, suicide is a 'selfish' and inconsiderate option. The views of other interested parties (e.g. loved ones) are often not considered. Attitudes towards life and death matters and how to deal with end-of-life decisions through euthanasia vary internationally and across Europe.

Wherever a sick person in perfect clarity of mind demands strongly that an end be put to an existence which has lost all meaning for them and wherever a committee of doctors sits for the purpose recognizes the unavailability of any other treatment, euthanasia should be granted (EC Human Rights Commission, 1991). A more recent case had the following ruling by the High Court, which redefined the meaning of withdrawal of treatment.

Box 9.5 Case: Burke v General Medical Council [2005] EWCA Civ 1003

A patient diagnosed with a degenerative brain disease effectively challenged the GMC guidelines for deciding on withdrawal of treatment for a patient diagnosed as being in a persistent vegetative state. According to The Times, 'the ruling reflects a shift from the medical profession and into the hands of patients. It also however forms part of a less welcome shift in power out of the hands of practitioners and into the hands of the courts' (The Times, 31 July 2004). The effect was to oblige the medical staff to continue with active (probably relatively expensive) treatment which some may see as futile, even though Mr Burke was considered to be in the terminal stages of life.

On appeal, the House of Lords and the European Court of Human rights held that doctors should not be expected to continue treatment of a patient (who suffered from muscle ataxia in this case) if in their judgement this was considered futile.

Do not attempt cardiopulmonary resuscitation orders

Here are some examples of the commonly used terms: 'do not resuscitate', 'do not attempt resuscitation', 'not for resuscitation', 'not for the call', 'not for 2222' or any other number assigned for cardiopulmonary arrest emergency calls. The Resuscitation Council outlines situations when resuscitation is considered futile (BMA, 2007). The first recorded attempt to administer resuscitation was around 800 BC in Elijah's attempt to give a child 'mouth to mouth' (King James' Version Bible, 2 Kings 4:34–35). Mouth-to-mouth resuscitation was first attempted as early as 1950. Cardiopulmonary resuscitation was not then used in hospitals except to 'prevent premature death in previously "fit" patients, who sustained a sudden cardiac or respiratory arrest' (Levack, 2002, p. 2). There are times when questions may be asked about the appropriateness of the use of cardiopulmonary resuscitation, especially when this is deemed futile due to a poor outcome prognosis – a quality-of-life issue.

Healthcare professionals need a theoretical moral framework, such as 'Principlism', to guide them in making ethical decisions when issues on end-of-life decisions may be related to a resuscitation status. There is debate as to whether a patient should be involved in decision-making related to their resuscitation status and whether every patient's permission should be sought for doctors to include a 'non-resuscitation' status in a patient's notes. This could be interpreted as withdrawal of treatment.

Box 9.6 Thinking point: case study

A 67-year-old cancer patient found out she had had a Do Not Attempt Cardiopulmonary Resuscitation (DNACPR) order written on her medical notes without her consent. The patient saw that her notes had a 'do not resuscitate' entry from a previous admission. She complained that she had not been consulted about this decision or options regarding whether she would like to be resuscitated. As it happened, the patient in question had a wish to be resuscitated in the event of a cardiac arrest: 'she was understandably distressed by this as no discussion had taken place with her or her next of kin', said a doctor (BBC News, 27 June 2000).

http://news.bbc.co.uk/1/hi/health/808206.stm

An inappropriate 'do not resuscitate' order may result in conflict and breach of trust between the patient, family members and healthcare professionals (Beigler, 2003). Owing to threats of litigation, modern healthcare practice may develop a culture of defensive medicine, assuming that prior to every death, cardiopulmonary resuscitation should be pursued. Professional bodies have issued the guidelines Decisions Relating to Cardiopulmonary Resuscitation, as an example of joint work by the British Medical Association (BMA), the Resuscitation Council (UK) and the Royal College of nursing (RCN). The BMA as well as related medical royal colleges and the RCN have all agreed on a code of practice (BMA, 1995) (see also the GMC's (2016) Guidance to Good Medical Practice).

There are changes to the guidelines. This means that the overall clinical responsibility for decisions about cardiopulmonary resuscitation including Do Not Attempt Cardiopulmonary Resuscitation (DNACPR) decisions lies with the most senior clinician as defined by local policy. This person may be a consultant, GP or suitably experienced senior or specialist nurse. This obviously may create ethical issues on decision-making and accountability especially when time is of the essence.

In England and Wales:

- You can plan ahead for this situation by choosing somebody who you want to be involved in future decisions if you are unable to take part. You do this by arranging to give them a "Lasting Power of Attorney" (LPA) for your health and welfare.
- The Court of Protection may also appoint a "Deputy" with similar powers.
- If, like many people, you do not have a LPA or Deputy, the health professional in charge of your care will make a decision about what is best for you, taking

into account your previously expressed wishes. They will ask your family or close friends for information about these. If you have no family or friends to ask, an "Independent Mental Capacity Advocate" may be asked to help.

(Resuscitation Council)

This provision does not extend to Northern Ireland, where clinicians are expected to consult family members if unable to establish the patient's wishes. In Scotland, however, a patient may have a representative or an advocate making decisions on their behalf in their capacity as the patient's 'Welfare Attorney'.

- The Sheriff may also appoint a "Welfare Guardian" with similar powers.
- If you do not have a Welfare Attorney or Guardian, the health professional in charge of your care will make a decision about what will benefit you, taking into account your previously expressed wishes. They will ask your family or close friends for information about these.

(Resuscitation Council)

It is obviously very different if this is an emergency. If there is no reason to believe that the patient is likely to have a cardiac or respiratory arrest it is not necessary to initiate discussion with the patient (or those close to patients who lack capacity) about CPR. If, however, the patient wishes to discuss CPR this should be attempted, unless the patient has capacity and states that they would not want CPR attempted.

- Decisions about CPR are sensitive and complex and should be undertaken by experienced members of the healthcare team and documented carefully.
- Decisions should be reviewed regularly and when circumstances change.
- Advice should be sought if there is uncertainty.

(BMA, 2007)

The Department of Health requires clinical areas to have in place resuscitation policies 'which respect patients' rights in place, understood by all staff and accessible to those who need them, and that such policies are subject to appropriate audit and monitoring arrangements' (NHS Executive, 2000, p. 1). Such a policy should be published locally for all interested parties.

It is important to involve family members in the decision-making (where possible to ascertain the patient's wishes); however, only the court may have the final decision on withdrawal of treatment. In cases where there is a diagnosis of persistent vegetative state (PVS) the state 'results from severe damage to the cerebral cortex, resulting in destruction of tissue in the thinking, feeling part of the brain. Patients appear awake but show no psychologically meaningful responses to stimuli and it is common for cerebral atrophy to occur. The condition is distinguished from a state of low awareness and the Minimally Conscious State (MCS) where patients show minimal but definite evidence of consciousness despite profound cognitive impairment' (BMA, 2016). The patient is required to have been in such a state for more than six months. It is the responsibility of the healthcare professionals to keep the family informed of any changes. The effect of any perceived or real shortcomings in the care of their loved ones may adversely affect them. Many would argue that the role of the healthcare professional is one of promoting rather than terminating life (Keown, 1997).

Where a service user lacks competence or capacity, healthcare professionals and the next of kin can agree to withdraw treatment or not to initiate new active treatment, provided this is in the patient's best interest (Section 2, Mental Capacity Act 2005). Competence may be specific to informed consent, which means that the user may be confused in some respects, though they may demonstrate an understanding of the benefits and risks related to the treatment. On withdrawal of treatment please see the decision in the Tony Bland case. When there is disagreement between healthcare professionals and family members, the matter should be referred to the courts for a judicial review. By carrying out inappropriate treatment there is a danger of raising the hopes of family members close to the patient without achieving much. The most difficult moment for healthcare professionals and family members is likely to be when a decision to withdraw treatment must be made. This has to be done when it is obvious that despite acute interventions, the patient is going to die, and the treatment is said to be futile. Winter and Cohen (1999) observe that there are difficulties in justifying the use of the term 'relatively futile' in respect of such treatment. It may be dangerous, as it introduces an unknown and potentially variable factor – namely the doctor's judgement (Winter and Cohen, 1999, p. 3). A clinical judgement may turn out to be wrong, as in the following case.

Box 9.7 Case: Glass v United Kingdom [2004] (application no. 61827/00)

The case followed the admission of a patient, a child who suffered from learning disabilities, who was in a poor state, suffering from a chest infection. He was represented by his mother as guardian, who sued the trust because doctors had made the decision to treat the patient and place a 'do not attempt resuscitation order' above his bed and had started a diamorphine pump. This was all done without consulting his mother. A physical fight ensued, during which several police officers and two doctors were injured. The patient's mother nevertheless wanted his treatment continued. The court held unanimously in favour of the patient on the basis that the trust had been in breach of Article 8 (right to respect for private life) of the European Convention on Human Rights and Fundamental Freedoms 1950.

The following case, considering the validity of DNACPR orders, also highlights this issue:

Box 9.8 Case: Re R (Adults: Medical Treatment) [1996] 31 BMLR 127

A 23-year-old man who was born with brain damage had multiple medical problems which included having developed epilepsy as a child. Unable to communicate, he appeared to be constantly in considerable acute pain. He was, however, conscious, having required constant care in a nursing home for the previous four years with weekend respite care, and he had been in and out of hospital with various ailments. There had been an agreement between the family and doctors that he should not be a candidate for active resuscitation. The trust, however, sought a declaration on withdrawal of treatment. It was held by Sir Stephen Brown that the 'do not resuscitate' order was lawful, on the basis that in cases where cardiopulmonary resuscitation was unlikely to succeed, this could be justified.

One leading case law in Scots law (*Law Hospital NHS Trust v Lord Advocate [1996] 2 FLR 407*) inclined towards a different approach in favour of withdrawal of treatment. However, the GMC's guidelines on withholding and withdrawing life-prolonging treatments (GMC, 2002, paragraph 16) require that, in the first place, 'doctors must take account of patients' preferences when providing treatment. However, where a patient wishes to have a treatment that in the doctor's considered view is not clinically indicated, there is no ethical or legal obligation on the part of the doctor to provide it'. This was updated in 2007 and is due for further update in 2014. Difficulties may arise when family members disagree with the decision to continue treatment, as illustrated in the following case.

Box 9.9 Case: W Healthcare NHS Trust v H [2005] I WLR 834

A nasogastric feeding tube for a 59-year-old MS patient fell out. The patient was conscious but had lacked mental capacity for decision-making, having been on tube feeding for five years prior to this. The family objected to the tube being reinserted. It was held by the court that in the absence of a valid advance directive, it was in the patient's best interest for the tube to be reinserted.

Persistent vegetative state (PVS)

One definition for PVS is

> A person who has lost cognitive neurological function, meaning that the upper part of the brain that controls the more sophisticated functions, such as speech, movement and thought, has died. People in PVS are able to breathe unaided as the lower part of the brain (the brain stem) is still functioning.
>
> (NHS Direct Online Health Encyclopaedia, 2002)

It is important to attempt to distinguish between PVS and a comatose state. In the case of the former, the condition is scientifically irrecoverable once the harm is done. If a patient is in a coma there is a chance of recovery. The Royal College of Physicians acknowledged that 'any diagnosis of PVS is not absolute but based on probability' (Royal College of Physicians, 1996, pp. 119–21). In the case of a patient in a PVS who may be on a ventilator, the withdrawal of treatment must be more formal, and guidelines set out by the BMA and the GMC should always be followed (see *Bolam v Friern Hospital Management Committee [1957] 1 WLR 582*). There may be difficulties in establishing the criteria, as PVS stems from the distinction between a 'brain stem' death, where there is loss of neurological functions and evidence of basic life, and a biological death (Campbell et al., 2005).

A patient who is being fed by artificial means may be considered alive only in the most basic of the biological or vegetative sense if they are deprived of brain function. It is believed that the true sense of death means that when this occurs, it is irrevocable and the functioning is irreversible (Campbell et al., 2005). The brain damage must be so severe that the condition cannot be reversed. Ongoing expensive treatment raises questions about how far medical science should go to sustain life for a 'brain dead' patient.

A patient is regarded as having been in PVS or a condition closely resembling PVS if this has persisted for at least six months. In England and Wales, a court order to withdraw treatment was expected to be sought for a review (BMA, 2003). On artificial nutrition and hydration for patients, new guidelines on nutrition and hydration require the doctor to follow the health and welfare attorney's decision, unless this is contrary to the patient's best interests (BMA, 2018).

Box 9.10 Thinking point

John, a 25-year-old single young man who was a successful professional footballer, suffered head and multiple injuries in a car crash, requiring an emergency admission to hospital. He was the only child of a middle-aged couple. He had undergone two surgical procedures to remove a blood clot following a sub-dural haemorrhage and returned to the intensive care unit. He had not made any significant improvement since the last operation and had in fact suffered from a stroke and resulting brain stem damage. Over the following week post-operatively, his general condition steadily deteriorated; the prognosis was poor, and his family was obviously devastated by the news.

A week later, the consultant physician responsible for John's care advised the parents that their son was not making any progress and that he was now in a PVS, having been an inpatient for the last six and a half months in the high dependency unit. The consultant discussed discontinuing treatment with the family, who were against this.

Consider the ethical and legal issues in the above scenario.

Living wills, advance decisions, statements and the right to choose

Living wills are the physical evidence of a patient's wishes should their condition deteriorate, and they are too incapacitated to indicate their wishes. Similar arrangements are now in place in England and Wales (Sections 24–26 of Mental Capacity Act 2005), following Scotland (Adults with Incapacity (Scotland) Act 2000), where a healthcare proxy document is used to describe either a living will or the full power granted to a proxy to make decisions on the patient's behalf. In the case of *Airedale NHS Trust v Bland [1993] 1 All ER 821 HL*, Lord Goff, at 872, in particular, said that the courts would reject the 'substituted judgment test', which means the court will not recognize any decision on the basis of informal arrangements for proxy decision-making.

Advance decisions to refuse treatment: general

> 24. (1) 'Advance decision' means a decision made by a person ('P'), after he has reached 18 and when he has capacity to do so, that if
> (a) at a later time and in such circumstances as he may specify, a specified treatment is proposed to be carried out or continued by a person providing healthcare for him, and
> (b) at that time, he lacks capacity to consent to the carrying out or continuation of the treatment.
>
> (Mental Capacity Act 2005)

Advanced statements are general statements of a person related to their preference for treatment: for example, a wish to be cared for in their own home at the end of their life. Such preferences, nevertheless, do not have the force of law. Healthcare professionals should, where possible, follow this; however it is not legally binding. They may only be used as an indication of treatment a patient may choose to decline, not as a basis for demanding certain forms of treatment. Some examples of patient choice may apply to individual choice based on religious or cultural preferences. It is always preferable to involve in decision-making as well as support next of kin and keep them informed. This includes family members, partners, wives or husbands or children.

Advance decisions, on the other hand, are a patient's formal instructions on their wishes to refuse certain specified treatment should their condition deteriorate. An advance refusal of treatment may be made by a person aged 18 or older with the necessary mental capacity to understand any medical, surgical or dental treatment or other procedure and is intended to remain in effect any subsequent time when they are without capacity to refuse consent.

The Law Commission report on mental incapacity (Law Commission, 1995) recommended acceptance of any advance 'refusals' of consent to treatment as well as the principle of patient autonomy. This recognizes human rights for patients and includes the right to accept or refuse treatment. Since the ruling in *Airedale NHS Trust v Bland [1993] 1 All ER 821 HL*, living wills have been recognized as evidence of 'the patient's wish' to limit or refuse treatment. Any will which is drawn up prior to a patient's deterioration must satisfy the above prerequisites, and for the will to have legal validity it must originate from a person who is of competent mind. The essential elements of a living will are similar to and have the force of an ordinary will in trust law. These were based on the BMA 1995 code of practice on advance directives (Dimond, 2002):

- full name,
- address,
- name and address of next of kin,
- whether advice was sought from health professionals,
- signature,
- date drafted and reviewed,
- witness signature,
- a clear statement of patient's wishes,
- name, address and telephone of nominated person.

(BMA, 1995; Dimond, 2002)

Since October 2007, living wills have been recognized in law (Mental Capacity Act 2005, with Sections 24–26). For an advance decision (previously known as directive) to be valid, the following conditions must be met:

- The advance directive (now decision) is made by a competent adult (18 years old and over).
- It is entered into voluntarily – the individual was not coerced into making the statement.
- The individual is sufficiently informed about the medical prognosis if the advance refusal is respected.

(Griffiths, 2008)

Patients may be admitted with a 'living will', which refers to either an advanced decision or an advanced statement. These will be valid only if the person has capacity at the time they were made. Capacity is now defined by the Mental Capacity Act 2005. This also provides for representation of a person who lacks capacity. There is now a legal requirement where there is no known relative or next of kin, for the appointment of an independent mental capacity advocate (IMCA). Their role is to represent and act on the service user's behalf. The clinician has a duty to consider the information provided by the IMCA.

An IMCA will only be involved if:

- The decision is about medical treatment provided by the NHS.
- It is proposed that the person is moved into long-term care of more than 28 days in a hospital or 8 weeks in a care home.
- A long-term move (8 weeks or more) to different accommodation is being considered, e.g. to a different hospital or care home.
- The IMCA service can be extended to specific situations if the local authority or NHS are satisfied that an IMCA would provide particular benefit, including:
- Care reviews regarding accommodation.
- Adult protection cases (even if the person who lacks capacity has family or friends.
- NB: An IMCA is not required if treatment is to be given under the Mental Health Act (1983).

(UKCEN)

Assessment of a patient's mental incapacity should be based on what is called the 'functional approach', based on the common law. This depends on whether at the time of decision the patient lacks the capacity for making. Capacity is presumed until proven otherwise and a patient should be empowered to be involved in decision-making (NHS Constitution, 2015). Where possible, patients need be encouraged and enabled to make informed decisions about their treatment on end of life (Department of Health, 2009).

Mental Health Act 1983 (Independent Mental Health Advocates) (England) Regulations 2008 provide for a similar independent mental health advocate (IMHA) representative role for a patient with mental health needs:

Independent Mental Health Advocates: conditions
6.—(1) A person may not act as an IMHA unless the conditions specified in paragraph (2) are satisfied.
(2) Those conditions are that the person referred to in paragraph (1)—
(a) has appropriate experience or training or an appropriate combination of experience and training;
(b) is a person of integrity and good character;
(c) is able to act independently of any person who is professionally concerned with the qualifying patient's medical treatment; and
(d) is able to act independently of any person who requests that person to visit or interview the qualifying patient.

In the absence of a living will, healthcare professionals are obliged to act in the patient's best interests in light of any evidence of the patient's previously expressed wishes (Section 4 of the Mental Capacity Act 2005). The case of Burke (discussed above) illustrates this point.

Incapacity may be temporary or permanent. Caring for an unconscious or PVS patient can be a stressful experience and a dilemma for the healthcare professional under whose care the patient is entrusted (Brazier, 2016). The American lawyer Louis Kutner is credited with the concept of 'living wills' in 1969, arguing that 'the legal trust established over property should be equally permissible and applicable to one's body' and emphasizing 'the importance of consent or withholding consent to treatment, whatever the prospect of recovery' (Kendrick and Robinson, 2002, p. 39). We have considered above how the law in the landmark Tony Bland case, *Airedale NHS Trust v Bland [1993] 1 All ER 821 HL [1993]*, paves the way for advance directives (now decisions).

If all the criteria for drawing up living wills are met, they should serve as valid evidence for giving a direction as to either what treatment to accept or what treatment to refuse (Nursing Times, 1999). Two consultants may give consent on behalf of an incapacitated patient in an emergency (Department of Health, 2001). Family members should be consulted only to establish the patient's best interests but not give consent on behalf of an incapacitated patient. If family members are not happy with a decision made by clinicians, they have no right under the law to overrule that decision but can seek a judicial review. Doctors, however, do not have to follow these directives if this is not in keeping with their training and their conscience; they are entitled to seek a second medical opinion if they disagree with the proxy. In an emergency, healthcare professionals are duty-bound to act in the patient's best interests. The basic principles of beneficence, non-maleficence and fairness are applicable. These are also part of articles of the Human Rights Act 1998.

The double effect doctrine and palliative care

Following the greater good principle or double-effect doctrine which accepts death as an unintended outcome, a positive act such as analgesia control (which is legitimate but may hasten the death of the patient) is lawful. Another example is termination of pregnancy where the mother's life may be at risk. This doctrine originates with Thomas Aquinas, who is credited with introducing the principle of 'the double effect' in his discussion of the permissibility of self-defence which is applicable to palliative care as the intent is to control pain, though effectively shortening life through respiratory depression.

- Killing one's assailant is justified, he argues, provided one does not intend to kill him.
- Aquinas observes that 'nothing hinders one act from having two effects, only one of which is intended, while the other is beside the intention'.

(Summa Theologica)

Accordingly, the act of self-defence may have two effects: one, the saving of one's life, which is the desired outcome, and the other, undesired, is the unfortunate killing of the aggressor. This principle was first developed in the following case;

The World Health Organization (WHO) defines palliative care as '... an approach which improves the quality of life of patients and their families facing life-threatening illness, through the prevention, assessment and treatment of pain and other physical, psychosocial and spiritual problems. The goal of palliative care is achievement of the best possible quality of life for patients and their families' (cited in Houses of Parliament Health Committee, 2004). Healthcare professionals have a duty of care in law and under the ethical principles of beneficence and non-maleficence to ensure that patients have adequate and appropriate pain control and not to overmedicate a patient. Their primary aim in the above case should be to achieve the right balance for pain as well as the timing of the level of pain control. Problems arise when time is clearly not to alleviate pain;

> ... death occurred earlier that it would have done from natural causes and was the result of the continuous administration of diamorphine, haloperidol, midazolam and hyoscine which had been prescribed to be administered continuously by a syringe driver for an undetermined number of days.
> (GMC100096, p. 163), Chapter 6: The General Medical Council)

If a patient is in pain, it may be difficult to ascertain their true needs if their declared request were an indication of a preference for 'euthanasia', saying they would like to 'end it all' or if, in fact, this may be an indication of their frustration and an expression of pain. It is possible that as soon as the pain is relieved, a patient will be a very different person and they may express a wish to be discharged home and/or to live a little longer. The nurse then faces a dilemma in ascertaining the patient's needs. It is possible that a patient's wish to 'end it all' may be motivated by unbearable pain and/or poor pain control or simply because they miss a loved one who has died before them. If the pain becomes intolerable, then they may see death as the only way out and a welcome relief.

Box 9.11 Case: R v Bodkin-Adams [1956] Crim LR (UK) 365

An elderly patient suffered a stroke, and the doctor (who happened to be a substantial beneficiary of the patient's will) decided to increase the opiate analgesic, and the patient died. It was held that he was not guilty of murder if the first objective of medicine, restoration of health, was successful and if the practice was backed by a responsible body of professionals.

It was held further by Lord Devlin that 'a doctor can do all that is proper and necessary to relieve pain and suffering, even if the measures he takes incidentally shorten life' as a side effect. The greater good principle would apply.

The courts in the UK are clear about their reluctance to extend the law on euthanasia demonstrating the dilemma when caring for a child, as is clear in the following case.

Staff decided not to give the child active treatment due to an expected short life expectancy.

Box 9.12 Case: A National Health Service Trust v D [2000] FCR 577

This case considered the right to resuscitation of a 19-month-old severely disabled child, and his life threatened from his illness. His doctors together considered that further treatment was not in his interests. They sought an order that in the event of future respiratory of cardiac failure, they should be free not to resuscitate him. His parents asserted that this infringed upon the child's human rights.

Held: The UK law position is that the child's interests are paramount. '[T]he court's clear respect for the sanctity of human life must impose a strong obligation in favour of taking all steps capable of preserving life, save in exceptional circumstances'. The court took the view that withholding life-prolonging treatment did not breach Article 2 of Human Rights Act 1998 and that the primary consideration should not be the views of the family members or friends of the patient. Any clinical decision on the course of action to be followed should be based on the patient's best interests. Mr Justice Cazalet observed that 'there does not appear to be a decision of the European Court which indicates that the approach adopted by the English courts in situations such as this is contrary to article 2'.

The court also acknowledged that the relevant consideration in treating the patient was not the doctors' views but the patient's best interest in relieving pain symptoms, albeit knowing that the side effect would be the hastening of death.

Crossing the Rubicon – towards a slippery slope

Torts law and Delict (Scots) law make no distinction between active measures and passive omissions, which may result in harm and breach of duty of care for a user or patient to have grounds for action in tort. It is relatively easy to establish a 'fiduciary relationship' between nurse and 'user' as this is based on trust. The case of *Donoghue v Stevenson [1932] UKHL 100* and subsequently the principle of law defined the duty of care applicable to nursing as to ensure that the patient is not harmed by their actions or omissions. The difficulty for a victim of clinical negligence is that they must meet the 'hurdles' before they can succeed. Difficulties may be posed in the clinical decision-making process and in setting a precedent when dealing with grey areas and the danger of 'crossing the Rubicon', hence the need for a judicial review by the courts, when a client lacks mental capacity or competence (see Tony Bland case: Airedale *NHS Trust v Bland [1993] 1 All ER 821 HL*; see Brazier, 2016). When conflicts arise, judges, who make decisions during judicial reviews seeking clarification on end-of-life decisions, must consider the morals of society, which shapes their own ethical considerations. The law is not always clear-cut, and a lot depends on whether there is some agreement with family members on whether to continue treatment. With any decision that allows the end of life, it is possible that some will see this as cheapening life, which must be preserved at all costs, while some may consider this a human right to be allowed to die with dignity. A recent supreme court case defined the law.

Box 9.13 Case: An NHS Trust and others (Respondents) v Y (by his litigation friend, the Official Solicitor) and another (Appellants) [2018] UKSC 46

Mr Y was an active man in his fifties when, in June 2017, he suffered a cardiac arrest which resulted in severe cerebral hypoxia and extensive brain damage. He never regained consciousness following the cardiac arrest. He required Clinically Assisted Nutrition and Hydration (CANH), provided by means of a percutaneous endoscopic gastrostomy, to keep him alive. The month after his cardiac arrest, Mr Y was admitted to the regional hyper-acute rehabilitation unit under the control of the first respondent NHS Trust so that his level of awareness could be assessed. In late September, his treating physician concluded that he was suffering from Prolonged Disorders of Consciousness (PDOC) and that even if he were to regain consciousness, he would have profound cognitive and physical disability, remaining dependent on others to care for him for the rest of his life. A second opinion was obtained in October, from a consultant and professor in neurological rehabilitation, who considered that Mr Y was in a vegetative state and that there was no prospect of improvement. Mrs Y and their children believed that he would not wish to be kept alive given the doctors' views about his prognosis. The clinical team and the family agreed that it would be in Mr Y's best interests for CANH to be withdrawn, which would result in his death within two to three weeks. The supreme court held that its decision will not be needed to withdraw treatment in agreed decisions.

Box 9.14 Thinking point

Peter, an 87-year-old man, is a retired accountant, in the advanced stages of lung cancer with secondary metastases in the spine. He was happily married for 60 years. Although not religious, he is known to have humanist sympathies, with no declared religion. He is now very drowsy with brief wakeful spells, when the pain becomes worse. He is unable to respond to conversation. He at times seems to be aware of the presence of his family and responds to his 86-year-old wife's voice. He had apparently informed one of his four sons, y, that he had no wish to live in view of his condition with unbearable pain. The son, claiming to represent his father's wishes, insists that antibiotic treatment for a chest infection should be stopped. Some family members, however, disagree and demand that because of their cultural and religious beliefs he should be treated aggressively until the very end (even if there is no clear evidence of a positive long-term prognosis). The patient himself is unaware of the ensuing dispute. The multi-disciplinary team consensus is in favour of keeping the patient pain-free and comfortable.

1 Consider the role of the nurse.
2 What are the patient's best interests, and what difference would a living will make in this case?

On the other hand, criminal law is very clear on liability and on the elements of murder. The *mens rea* (criminal intent) can be established as well as the *actus reus* (guilty act). This will not be the case when withdrawal is the only option, if it is agreed by the multi-disciplinary team that in the patient's best interests, further treatment would be futile, 'both medically and ethically, in the face of overwhelming disease' (Cohen, 1993, p. 52).

Box 9.15 Case: R v Shipman – [2004] QCA 171

Kathleen Grundy, an 81-year-old widow, who was an ex-mayoress of Hyde, respected and trusted her GP. She had followed him when he set up his solo practice and shortly before her death had even considered making a £200 donation to his practice fund. She was found dead on 24 June 1998. On Monday, 31 January 2000, the jury at Preston Crown Court convicted Dr Harold Shipman of murdering Mrs Grundy and 14 others.

Estimates of the number of people killed by Shipman range from a conservative 76 to over 1,000. It is possible that Shipman murdered more people than any other lone person in history.

How? The question that arises is 'How could this happen?', and there are no easy answers. Contributing factors might be the trust invested in doctors and healthcare professionals by their patients, and inadequate monitoring and poor systems of work within the health service and its professional associations.

Finally, it is useful to describe briefly how euthanasia has been received in other countries. Australia's Northern Territory passed the Natural Death Act 1988, which came into effect in July 1996, allowing euthanasia. It was in operation for less than a year (when four people were allowed to commit physician suicide) before being repealed by the federal government of Australia. In the United States, all states apart from Oregon do not allow physician- or other-assisted suicide. The Netherlands is of particular interest with more liberal views on euthanasia. It has strict guidelines to meet the following criteria:

(a) The request must come from the patient. It must, in addition be free and voluntary.
(b) This request must have been a considered and persistent one.
(c) The patient should be suffering intolerably ... there should be no prospect for improvement.
(d) The decision to end the patient's life must be one of the last resort having considered whether there is any less drastic alternative.
(e) The euthanasia must be performed by a doctor who has beforehand consulted with an independent doctor who has experience in the area of euthanasia.

(Davies, 1998, p. 352)

The Dutch practice of euthanasia was formalized by legislation in 2000 to allow both physician-assisted euthanasia and other assisted suicides. Official figures showed a significant increase (from 16 per cent to 41 per cent of deaths) in euthanasia between 1990 and 1995 (Hendin, 2002). The level of Dutch tolerance of euthanasia system has been criticized for failing to protect vulnerable patients and to address patients' choice and their right to autonomy, by failing to obtain proper and informed consent prior to euthanasia in more than 1,000 cases (Hendin, 2002). The worrying factor here is that it is almost impossible to tell the real number of such cases as this is difficult to monitor, and to establish doctors' compliance with the guidelines and monitoring can be difficult. Similarly, other European countries such as Switzerland and Belgium have followed suit in legitimizing physician-assisted euthanasia.

The Select Committee on Medical Ethics (House of Lords, 1993–94, paragraph 260; Walton Committee, 1994) drew a line on morality, which they felt at the time reflected the feelings of the majority of the UK public, and refused to extend the law by 'crossing the line which prohibits any intentional killing, a line which we think it is essential to preserve'. They suggested further that it was important that the move to block the legitimization of 'intentional killing' was seen 'as the cornerstone of law and the social relationships' (House of Lords, 1993–94). Where there is a lack of clarity or dispute, a judicial review should always be sought in order to safeguard patient rights. The law as it stands in the UK is based on the rule in *Airedale NHS Trust v Bland [1993]*, in which Lord Goff (at 870–1) observed that artificial feeding and hydration should only be discontinued when a patient's condition is deemed to be permanent, and discontinuing is in their best interests. He went on to demonstrate his dilemma in balancing continuing treatment against stopping:

> It is not lawful for a doctor to administer a drug even though that course is prompted by humanitarian desire to end his suffering, however great that suffering may be.
> Furthermore, there is a need for balancing the patient's needs for pain control and their interest in being put through what can only be seen as burdensome treatment, and so to cross the Rubicon which runs between, on the one hand, the care of the living patient and on the other hand, euthanasia actively causing his death, to avoid or to end his suffering. Euthanasia is not lawful at Common Law.
>
> *Airedale NHS Trust v Bland [1993]*

If physician-assisted suicide were lawful in the United Kingdom, there would be real difficulties for doctors in determining or ascertaining motivation for a patient's request or potential agreement to 'euthanasia', which could be linked to depression. A potential conflict of interest would be possible where family members would disagree with clinical judgements doctors could legally 'assist' the patient to die.

Physician-assisted suicide

It is difficult to establish the number of cases of euthanasia, although UK research involving general practitioners has suggested a figure of 584,791 deaths in England, Wales, Scotland and Northern Ireland. The most significant areas were alleviation of symptoms with possible life shortening (32.8 per cent) and non-treatment decisions (30.3 per cent). No voluntary euthanasia was recorded. Some have suggested that since its initiation as many as 453 people including 30 from the United Kingdom have been given assisted euthanasia through Dignitas, in Switzerland (LifeSite, 2005). The challenge facing organizations such as Dignitas is that it may not be easy to establish the patient's motive, before facilitating suicide, in that the motivation for ending life may be other than an intolerable suffering due to a medical condition and/or pain as in one case reported by Leidig (2005). Not so long before the issuing of the Director of Public Prosecutions guidelines in England and Wales, in 2009–10, 17 cases had been recorded by the police where complaints had been made about 'assisted suicides'; meanwhile, there were over 100 cases of Britons known to have ended their lives in Switzerland with assistance from Dignitas

(CPS, 2010). The DPP guidelines do not apply to Scotland, which follows its own criminal law system.

Following the ruling of the House of Lords, *R v DPP ex p Purdy [2009] UKHL 45*, the Director of Public Prosecutions (2010) aimed to clarify the law by issuing guidelines:

> The policy is now more focused on the motivation of the suspect rather than the characteristics of the victim. The policy does not change the law on assisted suicide. It does not open the door for euthanasia. What it does is to provide a clear framework for prosecutors to decide which cases should proceed to court and which should not. Difficulties remain in the interpretation of the guidelines, where there may be a need to balance interests of the patient and those of family members and society. The patient's best interests should be at the centre of decision-making. The difficulty is establishing those 'best interests' may be problematic, as it may be felt that the person asking to die may be under considerable pressure or indeed clinically depressed.

Box 9.16 The Director of Public Prosecutions (DPP) guidelines (updated 2018)

The DPP guidelines have been interpreted in the so-called 'locked-in syndrome' cases, for example the Tony Nicholson and Paul Lamb cases, and they have so far failed to persuade the courts to change the law. The first person was deceased at the time of the appeal but represented by his family members.

Lord Justice Toulson introduces the two cases (paragraphs 1–4):

These are tragic cases. They present society with legal and ethical questions of the most difficult kind. They also involve constitutional questions. At the invitation of the court the Attorney General has intervened. (Para 1)

Put simply, the claimants suffer from catastrophic physical disabilities, but their mental processes are unimpaired in the sense that they are fully conscious of their predicament. They suffer from 'locked-in syndrome'. Both have determined that they wish to die with dignity and without further suffering, but their condition makes them incapable of ending their own lives. Neither is terminally ill, and they face the prospect of living for many years. (Para 2)

Barring unforeseen medical advances, neither Martin's nor Tony's condition is capable of physical improvement. Although they have many similarities, there are some differences in their condition. There are also differences in the orders which they seek and the ways in which their cases have been presented.

Cases: Tony Nicklinson v Ministry of Justice, AM v Director of Public Prosecutions and Others, High Court (Administrative Court), 16 August 2012

Conclusion

Similar to healthcare professionals, judges may also face a dilemma in rulings on end-of-life decisions. There are often grey areas and complex clinical decisions, which are fraught with difficulties and with ethical implications. Some judges have wrestled with their own ethics or morality, and the dictum from the Bland case (above) summarizes this:

> The conclusion I have reached will appear to some to be almost irrational. How can it be lawful to allow a patient to die slowly though painlessly over a period of weeks from lack of food, but unlawful to produce his immediate death by a lethal injection, thereby saving his family from yet another ordeal? (Furthermore) I find it difficult to find a moral answer to that question. But it is undoubtedly the law.
> (Lord Browne-Wilkinson, Tony Bland v Airedale NHS Trust [1993])

Healthcare professionals, on the one hand, should act as representatives of their respective professional bodies and as advocates for vulnerable users. Occasionally, a conflict of interests may arise, as they wrestle with their conscience. The courts, on the other hand, have the opportunity to bring in changes by the back door by widening the interpretation of the legislation as intended by Parliament. The European Court of Human Rights may strike down any UK judgements that appear to contravene human rights legislation.

The role of ethics is to provide frameworks that are based on custom and human knowledge, which is fallible and has been subject to change at different times in history. Is it possible then that as a society we in the UK are becoming more and more indifferent to the value of human life and turning a blind eye to our innate conscience? As considered above, some philosophers, like Kant (1724–1804), believed that ignoring our 'categorical imperative', which he believed to be a moral compass, is wrong. An individual's choice to end their life, as opposed to preserve their life, could be immoral. The utilitarian view would make end-of-life decisions on the basis of usefulness to the majority in society rather than the best interests of the patient; thus, there is a possibility of rendering the concept of 'individual autonomy' redundant and meaningless and leaving some patients vulnerable. This could be seen as an easy way out rather than a last resort.

There is no clear evidence that in countries where euthanasia is legal the link between depression and requests for euthanasia is necessarily taken into consideration. Societal values that may conflict, internationally or even within a given society, are difficult to change overnight. There is so far no persuasive evidence to convince the public and the healthcare professional bodies in the UK that the interests of the patient would be best served by widening the category of patients eligible for euthanasia. So far, the UK Parliament does not support changing the status quo.

One ethical dilemma facing any healthcare professional involved in end-of-life decisions is that, even in the case of a patient who has the capacity to decide, they may never be able to say with certainty whether or not a request for 'euthanasia' is a cry for help or down to pressure from others.

A balance should be struck between the patient's interests and those of others, also taking into account the healthcare professional's own personal conscience and following professional guidelines (within the constraints of the law). There may be practical difficulties with family members, an informal representative, or a healthcare proxy, if, say, they themselves have vested interests in inheritance; if proven, such a motive may invite criminal prosecution. Attempts to change the law via a 'Patient Assisted Dying Bill' have so far failed. This would legalize euthanasia with a provision for opting out for conscientious objectors, as well a chance for a competent patient's considered decision. With no answers, the debate on end-of-life decisions goes on, and the moral dilemmas remain.

References

Adults with Incapacity (Scotland) Act 2000.

Airedale NHS Trust v Bland [1993] 1 All ER 821.

An NHS Trust and others (Respondents) v Y (by his litigation friend, the Official Solicitor) and another (Appellants) [2018] UKSC 46.

Aquinas T. Summa Theologica, II-II, qu. 64, art. 7. 1225–74. Available online at: http://www.newadvent.org/summa/3064.htm (accessed on 2nd October 2013).

BBC News. Patients must decide on resuscitation, 27 June 2000. Available online at: http://news.bbc.co.uk/1/hi/health/808206.stm (accessed on 14th December 2019).

Beauchamp TL, Childress J. *Principles of biomedical ethics*, 7th ed. New York: Oxford University Press, 2013.

Beigler P. Should patient consent be required to write a do not resuscitate order? *Journal of Medical Ethics* 2003; 29: 359–63.

BMA. Advance statements about medical treatment: Code of practice with explanatory notes. London: BMJ Publishing Group, 1995. Available online at: www.bma.org.uk/ap.nsf/content/withholdingwithdrawing (accessed on 2nd November 2019).

BMA. Decisions relating to cardiopulmonary resuscitation. A joint statement from the BMA, the Resuscitation Council (UK) and the RCN, London: British Medical Association, 2016. Available online at: https://www.bma.org.uk/news/media-centre/press-releases/2018/december/bma-and-rcp-publish-guidance-on-clinically-assisted-nutrition-and-hydration (accessed on 22nd December 2019).

BMA. Guidelines on treatment decisions for patients in persistent vegetative state. Revised December 2018. Available online at: https://www.bma.org.uk/news/media-centre/press-releases/2018/december/bma-and-rcp-publish-guidance-on-clinically-assisted-nutrition-and-hydration (accessed on 1st October 2019).

Bolam v Friern Hospital Management Committee [1957] 1 WLR 582.

Brazier M. *Medicine patients and the law*, 5th ed. London: Penguin, 2016.

Burke v General Medical Council [2005] EWCA Civ 1003.

Butterworths. *Butterworths' student statutes*, 2nd ed. London: Butterworths, 2000.

Campbell A, Gillett G, Jones G. *Medical ethics*, 4th ed. Oxford: Oxford University Press, 2005.

Cohen S. *Whose life is it anyhow?* London: Robson Books, 1993.

Crown Prosecution Service (2010). DPP guidelines on euthanasia. Available online at: https://www.cps.gov.uk/publication/assisted-suicide (accessed on 22nd November 2019)

Davies M. *Medical law*, 2nd ed. London: Blackstone Press, 1998.

Department of Health (2009). Guide to Consent. Available online at: https://www.gov.uk/government/publications/reference-guide-to-consent-for-examination-or-treatment-second-edition (accessed on 22nd November 2019).

Dimond B. *Legal aspects of pain management. British Journal of Nursing monograph*. Dinton: Quay Books, 2002.

Director of Public Prosecution (2010). Policy for prosecutors in respect of cases of encouraging or assisting suicide. Available online at: http://www.cps.gov.uk/publications/prosecution/assisted_suicide_policy.html (accessed on 10th October 2019).

Donoghue v Stevenson [1932], AC 532.

Dorland's Illustrated Medical Dictionary. The Shipman Inquiry. Available online at: https://www.dorlandsonline.com/dorland/home (accessed on 5th October 2019).

EC Human Rights Commission (1991). *Quoted by the Church of Scotland. Social work euthanasia, a church perspective*. Edinburgh: St Andrews Press, 1995.

Elford RJ. *The ethics of uncertainty*. Oxford: One World, 2000.

General Medical Council (2002). Withholding and withdrawing life prolonging treatments, paragraph 16. Available online at: www.gmc-uk.org (accessed on 20th August 2013).

Glass v United Kingdom [2004] (application no. 61827/00)

General Medical Council, 2010, in RCGP, 2012.

Griffiths J. (2008) Ethical considerations on the ICU. Available online at: https://www.anaesthesiauk.com/article.aspx?articleid=100889 (accessed on 23rd December 2019).

Hendin H. (2002). *Practice versus theory, the Dutch experience.* Houston: International Association for Hospices and Palliative Care. Available online at: https://hospicecare.com/policy-and-ethics/ethical-issues/essays-and-articles-on-ethics-in-palliative-care/euthanasia-and-physician-assisted-suicide-are-they-clinically-necessary-or-desirable/ (accessed on 10th November, 2019).

Houses of Parliament Health Committee (2004). Palliative care. Available online at: www.publications.parliament.uk/pa/cm200304/cmselect/cmhealth/454/454.pdf (accessed on 15th November 2019).

Kant I. *Fundamental principles in metaphysics of morals.* New York: Liberal Arts Press, 1785.

Kendrick K, Robinson S. *Their rights, advance directives and living wills explored.* London: Age Concern, 2002.

Keown J. *Euthanasia examined, ethical clinical and legal perspective.* Cambridge: Cambridge University Press, 1997.

Kubler-Ross E. *On life after death.* Berkeley, CA: Celestial Arts, 1991.

Law Commission (1999). The Law Commission report on mental incapacity. LC231. Available online at: www.lawcom.gov.uk (accessed on 2nd December 2012).

Law Hospital NHS Trust v Lord Advocate [1996] 2 FLR 407.

Leidig M. Dignitas is investigated for helping healthy woman to die. *BMJ* 2005; 331: 1160.

Levack P. Live and let die? A structured approach to decision making about resuscitation. *British Journal of Anaesthesia* 2002; 89: 683–86.

LifeSite (2005). Swiss euthanasia group Dignitas opening British office. Available online at: https://www.lifesitenews.com/news/swiss-euthanasia-group-dignitas-opening-british-office (accessed on 13th June 2019).

Medical Dictionary. Available online at: https://medical-dictionary.thefreedictionary.com/death (accessed on 2nd December 2019).

Mental Capacity Act 2004, section 4.

Mental Capacity Act 2005.

Mental Capacity Act 2005 sections 24–26.

Mental Health Act 1983 Mental Health Act 1983 (Independent Mental Health Advocates) (England) Regulations 2008.

Mental Health Act 2007.

Mental Health (Care and Treatment) (Scotland) Act 2003.

Morgan P, Lawton P. *Ethical issues in six religious traditions.* Edinburgh: Edinburgh University Press, 1996.

Natural Death Act 1983 [ceased] Repealed by Sch 3 cl 1(a) of Consent to Medical Treatment and Palliative Care Act 1995 on 30.11.1995.

NHS Direct (2002). Online Health Encyclopaedia. Available online at: NHS Direct (2002). Online Health Encyclopaedia.

NICE (2017). End of life care for adults, Quality Standard (QS13). Available online at: https://www.nice.org.uk/guidance/qs13/chapter/Introduction-and-overview (accessed on 21st November 2019).

NHS Constitution (2015). Available online at: https://www.gov.uk/government/publications/the-nhs-constitution-for-england (accessed on 6th November 2019).

NHS Executive. *Resuscitation policy.* HSC 2000/028. London: Department of Health, 2000.

NHS Trust v Bland [1993] 1 All ER 821 HL.

Nursing Times. *Nursing Times essential guides: Living wills.* London: EMAP Healthcare, 1999.

Pretty v the United Kingdom (European Court of Human).

R v DPP ex p Purdy [2009] UKHL 45.

Re R (Adults: Medical Treatment) [1996] 31 BMLR 127.

Re T (Adult: Refusal of Medical Treatment) [1992] 4 All ER 649, CA.

Regina v Cox [1992] 12 BMLR 38.

R v Shipman – [2004] QCA 171.

Resuscitation Council. Resuscitation Guidelines, Available online at: https://www.resus.org.uk/dnacpr/do-not-attempt-cpr-model-forms/ (accessed on 4th October 2019).

Select Committee on Medical Ethics (Walton Committee, 1994; House of Lords, 1993–94, paragraph 260). Available online at: http://www.lawcom.gov.uk/app/uploads/2015/04/lc231.pdf (accessed on 30th November 2019).

The Shipman Inquiry Report, Available online at: https://www.gov.uk/government/publications/overview-of-the-governments-action-programme-in-response-to-the-recommendations-of-the-shipman-inquiry (accessed on 1st October 2019).

Suicide Act 1961, Section 1.

Suicide Act 1961, Section 2(1).

Summa Theologica, II-II, qu. 64, art. 7. Whether it is unlawful to kill any living thing? Available online at: http://www.newadvent.org/summa/3064.htm (accessed on 6th September 2019)

Teichman J. *Social ethics, a student's guide.* Oxford: Blackwell Publishers, 1996.

UKCEN. The role of the mental capacity advocate. Available online at: http://www.ukcen.net/education_resources/mental_capacity/the_role_of_the_mental_capacity_advocate (accessed on 20th December 2019).

Tony Nicklinson v Ministry of Justice, AM v Director of Public Prosecutions and Others, High Court (Administrative Court), 16 August 2012.

Viney C. A phenomenological study of ethical decision-making experiences among senior intensive care nurses and doctors concerning withdrawal of treatment. *Nursing in Critical Care* 1996; 1: 182–87.

W Healthcare NHS Trust v H [2005] I WLR 834.

Winter B, Cohen S. Withdrawal of treatment. ABC of intensive treatment. *BMJ* 1999; 319: 306–8.

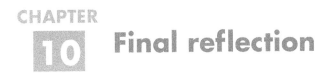

10 Final reflection

Chapter outline

Introduction

On a closing note, this chapter aims to present a summary of the key issues raised and to provide the reader with an opportunity for reflection by evaluating the development and impact of bioethics and human rights and the legal frameworks on care decisions. When human rights emerged, they were associated with the United Nations' Universal Declaration of Human Rights 1948. The impact of care decisions by the legal framework, and possibly morality, is inevitable. Legislating alone, however, may not be sufficient to prevent catastrophic cases of breaches of safety and abuse of patients at risk when things went wrong. Questions may need to be asked questions on how and why this may have happened. Examples include the R v Shipman case, the Mid Staffordshire case followed by the Francis Report (2013) and the more recent Gosport Memorial Hospital Case (2018), in which those at risk came to harm at the hands of healthcare professionals, the very people who they trusted. How could this have happened?

If there is a systems failure, this may be an indication that polices which are in place need reviewing and improving as this may mean that they are not effective enough. Unfortunately, due to human factors no guarantee can ever be given in order to ensure the safety of vulnerable people who may be at risk. Morality or ethical principles play a part in determining human conduct.

Paternalism vs. patient-centred care

Morals of a given society may also affect ethical standards expected of nurses and how they care for patients; nevertheless, the law must prevail, hence the limited reference to ethics in this final chapter. Professional codes of conduct should reflect the values of any given society and also make a positive impact on the quality of care delivered. The National Health Service (NHS) Plan (2000) had aimed to improve the patient's welfare through the following principles:

- Redress over cancelled operations
- Patients' forums and citizens' panels in every area
- New national panel to advise on major reorganization of hospitals
- Stronger regulation of professional standards

How far has nursing come in order to meet these expectations?

It could be argued that for doctors the now largely obsolete or updated Hippocratic Oath's 'most basic principle was that a doctor must always cure patients, but never harm them' (Science Museum, 2013). This had aimed to underpin the biomedical model of care (which preferred to focus on restoration of a patient's biological functioning) but not so much the psychosocial aspect, giving a patient their own individuality and autonomy. Some medical schools worldwide no longer require doctors to swear the Hippocratic Oath; rather, they adopt some of the principles in their own codes of practice.

Patient preferences of a paternalistic model were supported by research by Arora and McHorney (2000), who reported that, given the choice, 69 per cent of patients preferred to leave decision-making to their doctor (and presumably the nurse). It is possible that a paternalistic decision-making (carried out by doctors or nurses) could leave vulnerable patients open to abuse by a few healthcare professionals. From a paternalistic perspective it could nevertheless be argued (albeit fallaciously) that the caring relationship could be based on factors such as absolute trust or fear and conversely the patient's vulnerability. This would assume that the clinician always knows what is best for their patients. This model does not leave room for patient engagement. In nursing, Florence Nightingale, as the founder of modern nursing, recognized the principles of ethics:

> It may seem a strange principle to enunciate as the very first requirement in a hospital that it should do the sick no harm.
>
> (Florence Nightingale 1860–1920)

The NHS Constitution (2015) required patients to be at the heart of decision-making. This will be reviewed every ten years.

Updated policy (and presumably) litigation may have changed a previously perceived view of benevolence for 'grateful' patients who would not be expected to assert their rights and be 'difficult' by asking questions or complaining. This could have been based on a 'mystical' healthcare profession which was revered if not feared by the patient. Patients today are now generally more questioning – and rightly encouraged to do so. Litigation is more a reality, and things are very different, with the patient being expected to be involved in decisions about their own care. This would mean that the ethical principles such as patient autonomy and informed consent are respected. In a paternalism model, there was no room for a partnership with patients concerning decisions about their own treatment. Paternalism was synonymous with blind 'trust' in doctors and other healthcare professionals such as nurses. The problem, however, was that without any guarantees of patients' rights, that trust could be breached and eroded when making unitary clinical decisions.

Human factors: when something goes wrong

The modern view of this relationship needs to consider the patient's holistic needs and sees nursing as being now based on

> the use of clinical judgment in the provision of care to enable people to improve, maintain, or recover health, to cope with health problems, and to achieve the best possible quality of life, whatever their disease or disability, until death.
>
> (Royal College of Nursing 2003)

Most patients are now more aware of their human rights and litigation is a reality. It may be more difficult for healthcare professionals to safeguard a vulnerable patient who may lack mental capacity for decision-making. Nursing has come a long way and should provide holistic treatment or care for the user. Peplau's vision may now be realized as she defined nursing as a 'human relationship between an individual who is sick, or in need of health services, and a nurse specially educated to recognize and to respond to the need for help' (Peplau, 2004, p. 6). Where the law is unclear the nurse must always consult senior professional colleagues and the multi-disciplinary team in acting 'in the patient's best interests'.

Modern nursing has emerged as an autonomous profession in partnership with medicine. We have moved away from a largely dependent profession subservient to medicine, thus reinforcing a notion that only doctors were qualified to make decisions on treatment – patient or multi-disciplinary involvement was not considered important. In the past, the doctor played the crucial if not exclusive decision-making role while leaving nurses to carry out the doctor's orders. In the paternalistic model, the patient, on the other hand, was probably not expected to voice any opinion or to be involved in decision-making. Before the Human Rights Act 1998, patients' rights may not have been recognized. Human rights were in danger of being ignored on the basis that the doctor knew what was best for their patients. Today's nurses are increasingly taking on medical (extended) and autonomous roles, with increased levels of accountability.

The emergence of modern medical science in the Western world also meant the development of treatment into hitherto unknown territory. An often-cited landmark American case on human rights, which, though persuasive, is not authoritative in the UK, defined a patient's common law and human right to self-determination:

> Every person of adult years and sound mind has a right to determine what shall be done with his own body.
>
> (Schloendorff v Society of New York Hospital
> 211 NY 125; 105 NE 92 [1914])

Since the implementation of the Human Rights Act (HRA) 1998 (in October 2000), patients have become increasingly aware of their human rights. Although it may not necessarily be linked, there has been an increase in complaints with the UK becoming a more litigious society. In 2005–06, there were 5,697 claims of clinical negligence and 3,497 claims of non-clinical negligence against the NHS, a small increase on the previous period, with £560.3 million having been paid out for clinical negligence claims for the same period (NHS Litigation Authority, 2007). The NHS Litigation Authority, which also monitors risk assessments claims while providing indemnity insurance for healthcare providers' organizations, with responsibility for the Clinical negligence

Scheme (CNST), Liabilities to Third Parties (LTPS) and Property Expenses Scheme (PES), received 10,129 clinical claims in 2012–13, which was a rise of 10.8 per cent on the 2011–12 period. Figures and this amount reflected a total of £46.9 million. The funding from the CNST does not include Existing Liabilities Scheme (directly funded by the Department of Health) and covers claims for incidents which took place before the 1 April 1995. In Scotland, clinical claims are reported to have shown an average of £35.6 million since 2009 (Herald Scotland, 2013).

More recently, 'between 2006/07 and 2017/18, clinical claims payments quadrupled, from £0.4 to £2.2 billion, with the number of reported claims doubling from 5,400 to 10,600 over the same period'. NHS resolution (2018).

Fundamental human rights

Human rights as provided in Schedule 1 of the Human Rights Act 1998 were the embodiment of the European Convention on Human Rights 1950, which originated from the Universal Declaration of Human Rights 1948, which was a declaration of the United nations on 10 December 1948. The UK, in 1953, was one of the first countries to ratify the European convention, although this was not legally enforceable in UK courts until the passing of the HRA 1998. The statute took effect from October 2000.

The basic tenets of human rights are found in the HRA 1998, Schedule 1 (2013), and only those relevant to health care are identified, with some examples of their application to case law below. The articles of human rights (2–14) and only the relevant ones which are applicable to healthcare practice will be identified here, with one or two examples below.

> Article 2: Right to life.
> 1 Everyone's right to life shall be protected by law. No one shall be deprived of his life intentionally save in the execution of a sentence of a court following his conviction of a crime for which this penalty is provided by law.
> Article 3: Prohibition to torture.
> No one shall be subjected to torture or to inhuman or degrading treatment or punishment.

This article has often been relied on, with allegations of its breaches where poor care is identified with an example in the leading case which went to the European Court of Human Rights (ECHR).

Box 10.1 Case: McGlinchey et al. v the United Kingdom, application no. 50390/99, judgement of 29 April 2003

A woman known to have a heroin addiction (and also suffering from asthma) was sentenced to four months for a crime and subsequently imprisoned. While an inmate, she suffered severe heroin withdrawal symptoms, which included nausea, vomiting and weight loss. She was seen by a doctor, who on her arrival saw the patient and advised the nursing staff to monitor her symptoms.

Nevertheless, her condition deteriorated over the weekend. During this time, nursing staff did not call a doctor, nor did they request for the woman to be transferred to a hospital. The following Monday morning she collapsed and required emergency admission to hospital, where she died.

It was held by the ECHR that the prison service was in breach of article 3 of HRA 1998 due to its failing to take appropriate steps to treat the prisoner's condition and relieve her suffering, and that they had failed to act sufficiently quickly to prevent the worsening of her condition.

This related to poor treatment decisions.

Article 5: Right to liberty and security. This may apply to detention unless this is under the Mental Act provisions or legitimate imprisonment.

Article 8: Right to respect for private and family life. This focuses on dignity and the patient's right to autonomy.

Article 14: Prohibition of discrimination. This may fall under the umbrella of the *Equality Act 2010, Articles*

Aspects of law and human rights can be described as absolute, limited or qualified (Department of Constitutional Affairs, 2006). To reinforce the classification of these articles please revisit the analysis in Chapter 1. Users with capacity should be allowed to make decisions which have an effect on their own treatment as well as their lives, especially those with continuing care needs (NHS Constitution, 2015).

Examples of public authorities who come under the jurisdiction of the HRA 1998 include local authorities, care commissioning groups, NHS trusts, or health boards, the police, prison and the Immigration Service. In reality, there are always difficulties for the patient in identifying evidence where their welfare is endangered by healthcare professionals' conduct. Most patients receiving health care are vulnerable and may lack physical or mental capacity. Patients may not have the energy to ensure that their rights are honoured and to fight against infringement of these rights, when recovery should be their primary concern.

The end of the Second World War brought to the forefront the issue of human rights and how best they should be safeguarded, in light of those who had perished because of the abuse of human rights. The Declaration of Human Rights 1948 in Geneva had recognized the need for protection of human rights in general, but especially had vulnerable people such as patients in mind. Owing to their physical and mental condition, many patients may fall into this category. Any person who is deemed to be a victim of a breach of human rights may bring an action under the articles of the European Convention on Human Rights 1950, HRA 1998. UK courts have a duty to apply this legislation, but a victim has the right of appeal to the European Court of Human Rights or they may lodge their case there instead if they so wish. It is recognized that the HRA has so far not managed to create a consensus of the law in specific areas (Mullally, 2006). What it has done is to generate a database of case law, which will be useful for victims of human rights' abuse. This resource will therefore facilitate the process of the application of human rights law (based on case law) in European Union member states.

The HRA 1998 has not diminished the substance of UK law in areas such as criminal law or employment law, but it has been able to benefit individuals in areas where interpretation of existing law lacked clarity or resulted in encroachment of human rights.

> The government remains fully committed to the European Convention on Human Rights, and to the way in which it is given effect in UK law by the Human Rights Act.
> (Department of Constitutional Affairs, 2006, p. 1)

The debate remains on why this key legislation does not apply to private organizations at present. Following Brexit, current legislation may be subject to review in future though it is difficult to see how a complete overhaul would be possible without compromising fundamental Human Rights.

Patient safety

The Nursing and Midwifery Council (NMC) Professional Code of Conduct and Ethics (2018) requires nurses to safeguard the patient's welfare as identified in the four themes. There is no doubt that that human rights' legislation has had a direct impact on national and NHS policy. Most people who are service users are vulnerable and may be at risk. Healthcare professionals should risk assess and, having identified the needs of patients, put into place a risk management plan with effective interventions.

Healthcare professionals should manage care of vulnerable people on the basis of risk management. Under the Health and Safety at Work Act (HASAWA) 1974, this means that any potential risks or hazards are reported and managed properly before a patient is harmed. This applies to both the employer and employee. Sections 2–5; for example,

> Section 2(1) duties of the employer
> employer has a duty to conduct his undertaking in such a way as to ensure, so far as is reasonably practicable, that persons not in his employment who may be affected by the conduct of his undertaking are not as a result exposed to risks to their health and safety.
> (Section 3(1) of Health and Safety at Work Act 1974)

Furthermore, on ensuring the health, safety and welfare of employees while at work) and employee:

> Section 7(a–b) It shall be the duty of every employee while at work:
> (a) To take reasonable care for the health and safety of himself and others who may be affected by his acts or omissions at work.
> (b) To co-operate with his employer or any other person, so far as is necessary, to enable his employer or other person to perform or comply with any requirement or duty imposed under a relevant statutory provision.
> (Health and Safety at Work Act 1974)

The National Patient Safety Agency (NPSA) was established by the UK government in July 2001 for the purposes of coordinating the efforts of NHS trusts in the UK by reporting mishaps and problems affecting patient safety and thus allowing trusts to learn from any mistakes. Since 1 June 2012, its key functions for patient safety were taken over by the NHS Commissioning Board Special Health Authority. NHS Improvement has taken over the responsibility of the NSPA and uses the National Reporting and Learning System (NRLS) to collate national statistics into six monthly reports nationally and make recommendations for improving practice.

While the NMC regulates the professional conduct for nurses, the Care Quality Commission (CQC) now regulates the providers to ensure that quality of care and that national standards are being met. The Royal College of nursing, as well as being a professional body, also represents nurses as a trade union. The dual role was questioned by the Francis Report (2013) in respect of Stafford Hospital. Accountability should be at the centre of care and all managers and professionals should be answerable for their actions.

> Recommendation no 2. –
> Putting the patient first
> The patients must be the first priority in all of what the NHS does. Within available resources, they must receive effective services from caring, compassionate and committed staff, working within a common culture, and they must be protected from avoidable harm and any deprivation of their basic rights.
>
> (Francis Report, 2013, p. 87)

Taking the bigger picture on accountability means that since 2013, the Department of Health has held the NHS Commissioning Boards to account regarding improvements in health outcomes and corresponding performance indicators. The Health foundation (2013).

The evidence suggested that limited progress had been made in taking on board human rights in order to ensure patients' rights are respected and questions may still be asked, and as a society, we still have some way to go in recognizing patient's rights when caring for them. Common experiences of patients were cited as follows:

> Not enough involvement in decisions
> No-one to talk to about anxieties and concerns
> Tests and/or treatments not clearly explained
> Insufficient information for family/friends
> Insufficient information about recovery
>
> (Department of Health, 2001)

The NMC has issued guidelines for nurses and midwifes and nursing associates on raising and escalating concerns (NMC, 2019). Breach of patients' rights and abuse of vulnerable users within a domestic environment continue to be a concern for both children and adults, so the latest legislation to combat this is the Domestic Violence, Crime and Victims (Amendment) Act 2012 (Commencement) Order 2012, SI 2012/1432 (c. 54). The 2012 Act extends the offence of causing or allowing the death of a child or vulnerable adult in section 5 of the 2004 Act ('the causing or allowing death offence') to cover causing or allowing serious physical harm (equivalent to grievous bodily harm) to a child or vulnerable adult ('the causing or allowing serious physical harm offence').

The majority of care that nurses and other healthcare professionals deliver is demonstrably positive and beneficial to the patient. However, occasionally a patient may experience a journey riddled with systematic failures, and their welfare may be adversely affected by dangerous practice, near misses or never events; the latter is defined:

Never Events NPSA 2009
Never Events are serious, largely preventable patient safety incidents that should not occur if the available preventative measures have been implemented by healthcare providers.

(NHS Improvement, 2016)

The year 2019 marks the 100th anniversary of the recognition of nursing as a profession: Ethel Gordon Fenwick, née Manson, a former matron of St. Bartholomew's Hospital in London, spent 30 years campaigning for the state registration of nurses, and this resulted in the Nurses Registration Act 1919. Today's nurses look very different and are more autonomous than ever. Autonomy means empowerment of the service user is real. This comes with autonomy and likelihood of litigation should things go wrong. Nightingale may have been criticized for promoting nurses as subservient to doctors.

Nevertheless, nurses must not forget the basics of Nightingale's theory which requires care to be patient-centred:

Patients are to be put in the best condition for nature to act on them, it is the responsibility of nurses to reduce noise, to relieve patients' anxieties, and to help them sleep.
As per most of the nursing theories, environmental adaptation remains the basis of holistic nursing care.

(Elsevier, Theory of Nightingale, 2012)

Since the inception of the NHS in 1946 it has become an established principle that all patients should receive free care at the point of delivery, with a mission to improve the quality of life through provision of universal health 'from the cradle to the grave'. The NHS Plan aimed to improve resources with 'the cash injection to boost capacity: 7500 more consultants; 2000 more general practitioners, 20 000 more nurses; 7000 more beds (particularly to boost intermediate care), investment in NHS facilities better healthcare provision by improving safety and recognising their human rights' (Department of Health, 2001). The latest NHS Long Term Plan (2019) means that there is some awareness of the need for an investment for the plan to work rather than short term disjointed strategies. This also included measures to:

- improve out-of-hospital care, supporting primary medical and community health services
- ensure all children get the best start in life by continuing to improve maternity safety including halving the number of stillbirths, maternal and neonatal deaths and serious brain injury by 2025
- support older people through more personalised care and stronger community and primary care services
- make digital health services a mainstream part of the NHS, so that in 5 years, patients in England will be able to access a digital GP over the next 10 years,

(NHS Long Term Plan, 2019)

The Kings Fund response to the long-term plan was

> This is an ambitious plan that includes a number of commitments which – if delivered – will improve the lives of many people. NHS leaders should be applauded for focusing on improving services outside hospitals and moving towards more joined-up, preventative and personalised care for patients.
>
> (The King's Fund response to the NHS long-term plan, https://www.kingsfund.org.uk/press/press-releases/ kings-fund-response-nhs-long-term-plan)

The success of the plan will depend on the political goodwill and commitment.

Final conclusion

An example of an amalgamation of anti-discriminatory legislation (which is relevant to care) is through the Equality Act 2010, and this should make it easier to outlaw discrimination. Another example of promoting patients' rights now means that patients with mental capacity should be given a sufficient degree of information to make an informed choice on treatment.

In the early days, Paternalism was seen as a by-product of medical science; we have nevertheless made progress in promoting the patients' rights. This belief may have been taken for granted as the norm not only by patients but also by doctors, nurses and other healthcare professionals. Paternalism meant that patients were not party to nor were they expected to question medical decisions on their own treatment. Even with good intentions, there was always room for their human rights to be compromised. A nurse must safeguard vulnerable patients' rights, especially those lacking capacity, by raising concerns with line managers and if necessary, escalating them (NMC, 2019), with the patient at the centre of clinical decision-making. Challenges for the future include an ageing population and people living longer. This means that there are now more demands on the service, considering the fact that there are also limited resources with cuts and austerity.

The development of IT means that there are better and more efficient treatment options for patients however, questions may be raised on accountability and ethics in decision-making.

Nurses will appreciate the significance and implications of their scope of practice and the benefits of autonomous practice as well as raised expectations when working in partnership with the patient, the multi-disciplinary team, as well as patient's next of kin and their friends and carers. With autonomy of practice, comes accountability. This means that a nurse should be able to justify decision-making and nursing actions while counterbalancing this with empowering their client. Accountability for nursing actions starts with the nurse's professionalism, as this is the basis of the nurse's relationship with the service user. Given that professionals may be entitled to consider 'accountability to themselves' (perhaps as they reflect on the efficacy and justification of their nursing decision-making and actions), it is also clear that individual morality alone may not suffice to justify or define especially when things go wrong. In order to protect the patient, there is a necessary requirement for formal professional regulation, and accountability must start with the NMC, through professional colleagues/

managers, the patient or user, the employer (under employment law terms of contract) and of course other branches of the law, such as health and safety law, criminal law or law of torts or delict.

With the majority of service users, everything goes according to plan and the aims of interventions are realized. Nurses should, nevertheless, acknowledge that, in spite of advances in medical science, evidence-based practice and the best intentions, human factors may prevail, and things may go wrong. In this category should be included neglect and inadequate care, which may impact adversely on patients' health and safety. If harmed, the patient or their representatives are entitled to seek recompense for personal injury, with damages being awarded in litigation for clinical negligence. Patients' rights should be realized and at the centre of any decision-making. Nursing actions should be based on evidence-based practice. When any nursing frameworks or care pathways are identified for use, the nurse must be able to justify their use and outcomes and demonstrate partnership with the user. They must always act in the patient's best interests.

References

Arora K and McHorney C. Patient preferences for medical decision making: Who really wants to participate? *Medical Care* 2000; 38: 335–41.

Department of Constitutional Affairs. *Making sense of human rights; a short introduction.* Crown, 2006. Available online at: www.dca.gov.uk (accessed on 30th April 2010).

Department of Health, The expert patient: a new approach to chronic disease management for the 21st Century (2001) para 1.7available online at: https://assets.publishing.service.gov.uk/government/uploads/system/uploads/attachment_data/file/250880/5103.pdf accessed on 6th May 2020.

Department of Health. *'NHS plan' a plan for investment.* London: NHS, 2000. Available online at: www.doh.gov.uk (accessed on 8th June 2019).

Elsevier, Theory of Nightingale (2012) Available online at: http://currentnursing.com/nursing_theory/Florence_Nightingale_theory.html (accessed on 23rd December 2019).

Francis Report (2013) Report of the Mid Staffordshire NHS Foundation Trust public inquiry. Executive summary. Available online at: http://www.midstaffspublicinquiry.com/ (accessed on 13th September 2019).

Herald, 25th February 2013 Revealed: £213m bill to NHS in negligence claims. February 2013. Available online at: https://www.heraldscotland.com/news/13093552.revealed-213m-bill-to-nhs-in-negligence-claims/ (accessed on 20th April 2020).

International Council for nursing (ICN Code). Available online at: https://www.icn.ch/sites/default/files/inline-files/2012_ICN_Codeofethicsfornurses_%20eng.pdf (accessed on 20th October 2019).

Mullally S. *Gender, culture and human rights: Reclaiming universalism.* Oxford: Hart Publishing, 2006.

National Health Service (NHS). The NHS plan, 2000. Available online at: https://navigator.health.org.uk/content/nhs-plan-plan-investment-plan-reform-2000 (accessed on 16th November 2019).

National Health Service (NHS). Constitution (2015) Available online at: gov.org (accessed 19th October 2013).

NHS Resolution (2018) NHS Litigation Authority Annual report and accounts 2017/18, available online at: https://resolution.nhs.uk/wp-content/uploads/2018/08/NHS-Resolution-Annual-Report-2017-2018.pdf (accessed on 6th May 2020).

National Health Service Litigation Authority (2007) Available online at: http://www.nhsla.com/home.htm (accessed 20th July 2008).

National Patient Safety Agency. Available online at: www.npsa.nhs.uk/ (accessed on 12th April 2010).

NHS Improvement (17 November 2016) Available online at: https://improvement.nhs.uk/resources/never-events-policy-and-framework-review-2016/

Nursing and Midwifery Council (NMC). *Code of professional standards of practice and behaviour for nurses, midwives and nursing associates*. London: Nursing and Midwifery Council, 2018.

Nursing and Midwifery Council (NMC). *Raising concerns guidance for nurses, midwives and nursing associates*, London: Nursing and Midwifery Council, 2019.

Peplau H. *Interpersonal relations in nursing: A conceptual frame of reference for psychodynamic nursing*. Basingstoke: Springer Publishing Company, 2004.

Royal College of Nursing. *Defining nursing*. London: Royal College of nursing, 2003. Available online at: www.rcn.org.uk (accessed on 1st February 2007).

Science Museum (2013) Available online at: http://www.sciencemuseum.org.uk/broughttolife/themes/controversies/hippocracticoath.aspx (accessed on 12th October 2019).

The NHS Long Term Plan (2019) Available online at: https://www.longtermplan.nhs.uk/wp-content/uploads/2019/08/nhs-long-term-plan-version-1.2.pdf (accessed on 21st December 2019).

Index

Note: To highlight case from other entries, we have entirely denoted in *italics*.

Milton Keynes UK
Ingram Content Group UK Ltd.
UKHW050117060424
440593UK00016B/164

9 780367 262457